Conscious Sedation in Gastroenterology

Conscious Sedation in Gastroenterology

A Handbook for Nurse Practitioners

Meg Skelly MDS(Lond), FDSRCPS, FDSRCS

*Senior Lecturer and Consultant in Dental Sedation,
Guy's, King's and St Thomas' Dental Institute*

and

Diane Palmer BSc(Hons), RN, PGCE

Lecturer in Nursing, University of Hull

SERIES EDITORS
Graeme Duthie MD, FRCS(Ed), FRCS
and
Diane Palmer, BSc(Hons), RN, PCGE

W

WHURR PUBLISHERS
LONDON AND PHILADELPHIA

© 2003 Whurr Publishers
First published 2003 by
Whurr Publishers Ltd
19b Compton Terrace, London N1 2UN, England and
325 Chestnut Street, Philadelphia PA 19106, USA

Reprinted 2003

British Library Cataloguing in Publication Data
A catalogue record for this book is available from the British
Library.

ISBN: 1 86156 266 7

Typeset by HWA Text and Data Management, Tunbridge Wells
Printed and bound in the UK by Athenaeum Press Limited, Gateshead, Tyne & Wear

Contents

Contributors

Duncan Bell MD, MSc, FRCP (Lond), FRCP (Edin) *Professor and Consultant Gastroenterologist, Sunderland Royal Hospital*

Carole Boyle BDS, MMedSci, FDSRCS, MFGDP(UK), MSNDRCSEd *Associate Specialist in Sedation and Special Care Dentistry, Guy's, King's and St Thomas' Dental Institute*

David Craig BA, BDS (Hons), MMedSci, MFGDP, Cbiol *Associate Specialist in Sedation*

Tom Cripps MB, BA, ChB, FRCA *Consultant Anaesthetist, Borders General Hospital*

John Elmore RGN, MSc(Clinical Nursing), DipNStudies(Critical Care) *Nurse Clinician, Whiston Hospital, Prescot, Merseyside*

Paul J Madigan RGN, DipEd, MSc *Nurse Consultant in Gastroenterology, Whiston Hospital, Prescot, Merseyside*

Sheila Mair RGN, DipN, BSc (Hons) *Gastroenterology Nurse Practitioner, Crosshouse Hospital, Ayrshire*

Diane Palmer BSc (Hons), RN, PGCE *Lecturer in Nursing, University of Hull*

Meg Skelly MDS (Lond), FDSRCPS, FDSRCS *Senior Lecturer and Consultant in Dental Sedation, Guy's, King's and St Thomas' Dental Institute*

Series Foreword

This series represents a significant addition to the nursing literature. The editors are respected experts and they have assembled a team of authors with the necessary experience and reputation to ensure the authority of each volume. From the stable of the prestigious specialist nurse endoscopy course at the University of Hull and based in the Hull and East Yorkshire Hospitals NHS Trust, this series will ensure that excellence will not be the preserve of these institutions.

Gastroenterology is an important field where nurses can develop and practise as specialist and advanced practitioners. The field extends from the inexplicable, such as irritable bowel syndrome, through the aetiological puzzle of inflammatory bowel disease, to life-threatening malignancies. Irritable bowel syndrome and inflammatory bowel disease both involve significant psychological morbidity and treatment in these areas is ripe for the development of nursing interventions such as counselling and behavioural therapies. Definitive diagnosis of inflammatory disorders and malignancies requires endoscopy, and this is an area where nursing makes a significant contribution through independent practice. Endoscopy is an invasive procedure which raises significant anxiety in patients and one where nurses are able to combine their psychosocial and technical skills. As such, nurses require well developed psychosocial skills – which are integral to nursing practice – and a deep knowledge of the anatomy and physiology of the gastrointestinal tract. The series will ensure that all nurses, particularly those who wish to practise in the field of gastroenterology, will have a sound foundation.

Roger Watson BSc, PhD, RGN, CBiol, FIBiol, ILTM, FRSA
Professor of Nursing, University of Hull

Preface

This book is one of a series of specialist texts for advanced nurse practitioners and specialists in gastroenterology. In addition to complementing the core text of the series *Core Skills for Nurse Practitioners*, this text has been written as a stand-alone volume. The chapter authors come from a wide spectrum of clinical specialties. All were invited to contribute to this book because of their extensive experience of conscious sedation, and all are well regarded in their disciplines. The majority are currently actively involved in the use of these techniques in their daily clinical practice.

Although primarily aimed at those working in the field of gastrointestinal endoscopy, we believe that this book will be a useful reference for both nurses and others involved in the clinical care of patients undergoing diagnostic or therapeutic procedures under conscious sedation in a variety of specialties. Each chapter covers a particular area of the practice of conscious sedation, subjects that are covered in more than one chapter being cross-referenced for easy reading. We hope that you will find this book both useful and interesting.

Diane Palmer and Meg Skelly
November 2002

Acknowledgement

We wish to thank Bernadette O'Riordan for her help in putting together the material for this book.

CHAPTER 1

History of sedation for endoscopy

Duncan Bell

It is useful to consider the historical development of endoscopy in order to appreciate the much more careful way in which we care for our patients today. In the early days of endoscopy, in both the USA and Great Britain, the drug doses used to sedate patients were often too high (Whitwam and McCloy, 1998; Freeman, 1999; Lazzaroni and Bianco-Porro, 1999). Combinations of benzodiazepines and opioids were frequently administered, with potentially fatal consequences (Bell, 1990; Whitwam and McCloy, 1998). We now know, however, that the best and safest endpoint for sedation comprises anxiolysis, amnesia and co-operation (Whitwam and McCloy, 1998), smaller doses than previously used thus being appropriate for the average patient:

> The sedationist should become adept at noticing the gentle relaxation of the patient. The 'white knuckles' of the anxious patient disappear as the patient begins to unclench his or her fists, the shoulders are lowered and the patient's facial muscles take on a calmer appearance and the legs rotate outwards.
>
> (Whitwam and McCloy, 1998)

Historical developments in endoscopy

The word 'endoscope' is derived from the Greek prefix *endo*, meaning 'within' and the word *scopein*, 'to observe'. In this chapter, we are concerned solely with fully flexible endoscopes such as gastroscopes, duodenoscopes, enteroscopes, colonoscopes and flexible sigmoidoscopes, but it should be remembered that endoscopy also employs rigid endoscopes such as laparoscopes, in which the optical system is totally different. James Le Fanu's book *The Rise and Fall of Modern Medicine* (Le Fanu, 1999) contains an excellent section on the work of Harold Hopkin and Basil Hirschowitz, leading to the development of fibreoptic endoscopes. The same book also provides a fascinating account of the discovery of the phenothiazines and minor tranquillizers such as diazepam.

It is not generally appreciated that Harold Hopkin – then a lecturer in physics at Imperial College, London – not only solved the problem of the fibreoptics of flexible endoscopes in 1954, but 5 years later also developed the Hopkin rod-lens system, which improved the quality of the laparoscopic image 80-fold. The British Society of Gastroenterology (BSG) makes an annual award of the Hopkin's Endoscopy Prize for the best research on an endoscopy-related topic. Up until his death, Hopkin would write personally to the winners, congratulating them and inviting them to explain in more detail their contribution to endoscopy and its importance. Neither flexible nor rigid endoscopy could have progressed to today's standard without this brilliant man's work. I agree with Le Fanu (1999) that it was totally unfair for him not to receive a Nobel prize in recognition of these two enormous contributions to medical science.

The story is said to have started back in 1951 at a dinner party in which Harold Hopkin met and subsequently engaged in conversation the St George's Hospital gastroenterologist Hugh Gainsborough (Le Fanu, 1999). Gainsborough complained that the gastroscopes then available were most inadequate: even the latest and most sophisticated semi-flexible gastroscopes required considerable expertise to use, and the poor patient suffered considerable discomfort during the procedure, which was likened to a sword-swallowing exercise. Furthermore, Hopkin was informed that the gastroscope's field of vision was severely limited, causing several 'blind spots' in both the cardia and fundus of the stomach, as well as in the first part of the duodenum. Gainsborough told Hopkin that it was therefore all too easy for the endoscopist to miss important pathology; what was required was clearly a gastroscope whose tip could be manipulated in several directions so that the entire lining of the stomach could be reliably visualized.

Hopkin was, as an optical physicist, aware that glass-blowers in Ancient Greece and Renaissance Venice had constructed beautiful objects made of thin cylinders of glass along which light could be conducted from a lamp underneath, with spectacular effect. He was also well aware of the experiments carried out at the Royal Society in London by John Tyndall in 1870, in which it was shown that light could be transmitted along the thin, curved path of a stream of water flowing from a small hole in the side of an illuminated vessel of water (Le Fanu, 1999). Hopkin speculated that if tens of thousands of very narrow flexible glass fibres were collected in a bundle, they should be able to transmit light around corners. Furthermore, the image of what was illuminated at the other end should be transmitted back up the fibre bundle to be viewed by the observer. The results of his 3 years' work were published in the journal *Nature* early in 1954.

As a physicist, Hopkin himself could not apply the fibreoptic principle to medical endoscopy; this was left to Basil Hirschowitz, a South African gastroenterology research fellow then working at the University of Michigan, USA (Le Fanu, 1999). Hirschowitz, like Gainsborough 3 years before him, was frustrated at the poor optics of the then 'state-of-the-art' gastroscopes. On reading Hopkin's paper on fibreoptics, Hirschowitz flew to London to meet the great man and see his prototype instrument. The important thing from Hirschowitz's point of view was not that the instrument was just 1 foot in length and thus unsuitable for practical use, but rather that the optical definition was excellent. Hirschowitz returned to America and proceeded to turn Hopkin's idea into the first practical flexible gastroscope.

A great deal of credit for the final success of the venture must go to Hirschowitz's collaborator Larry Curtis, who solved the problem of light jumping from one glass fibre to the next (so-called 'cross-talk') by producing glass-coated glass fibres. He did this by melting a rod of optical glass inside a tube of lower refractive index glass and pulling the two together into a thin composite fibre. Hirschowitz finally knew beyond all doubt that he was 'on to a winner' when one of Curtis's composite fibres was used to conduct a white spot of light 30 feet from one room to the next (Le Fanu, 1999).

Within 6 weeks, the first fully flexible gastroscope had been produced, some 200 000 fibres having to be orientated so that the two ends were in exact relation, forming a so-called 'co-axial bundle'. Having first swallowed the new instrument himself, Hirschowitz looked around for a suitable patient. Within a week, he had endoscoped the wife of a dental student and located a duodenal ulcer. The illumination of the stomach was a least two and a half times better than with the then-conventional semi-flexible gastroscope, and the whole of the gastric lumen could be easily visualized. Thus, in 1955 the semi-rigid gastroscope became obsolete overnight.

What subsequently happened in the way of a veritable explosion of interest, ideas and new endoscopic techniques is outside the brief of this chapter. Landmark gastrointestinal events, however, include the first description of endoscopic sphincterotomy in 1971, colonic snare polypectomy in 1973 and the introduction of video-endoscopes in the mid-1980s. The rapid growth of gastrointestinal endoscopy is well illustrated by the British experience. When I qualified in 1968, there were fewer than 2000 upper gastrointestinal endoscopies being performed per year in the whole of Great Britain (Salmon, 1974). In contrast, about 1% of the UK population now has an oesophagogastroduodenoscopy (OGD) in any given year, making about 550 000 examinations per year. It is sobering to look at figures reported from the 87 centres in the British Isles carrying out fibreoptic endoscopies between 1968 and 1972, which show that the number of colonoscopies carried out in 1969, 1970, 1971 and 1972 was 4, 80, 247 and 827 respectively (Salmon, 1974). The first 71 cases of endoscopic retrograde cholangiopancreatography (ERCP) were performed in 1971, with 401 cases in the following year (Salmon, 1974). In comparison, our own endoscopy unit in Sunderland, which covers a population of approximately 330 000, carried out about 4500 OGDs, 1000 colonoscopies, 950 flexible sigmoidoscopies and 300 ERCPs in 1999.

Safety record for endoscopy

Before discussing the sedation and safety aspects of endoscopy, it is important to understand a bit more about the development of early endoscopy units and the 'training' of the early medically qualified endoscopists. Like Topsy, endoscopy just grew! In the early 1970s and 80s, there was little in the way of funding for gastrointestinal endoscopy. Some endoscopy lists were undertaken by general surgeons, often in main theatres with an anaesthetist present, whereas others were carried out by physicians, often in day theatres, outpatient departments, side wards or any old room available in the hospital.

Many of the consultants in charge of gastroenterology units in the late 1960s and early 70s simply purchased endoscopes and, without any formal training whatsoever, started using the equipment – or worse still just left their junior staff to 'get on with it'. Although doctors such as Peter Cotton at the Middlesex Hospital and Christopher Williams at St Mark's rapidly established 'centres of endoscopic excellence' in the 1970s, this was very much the exception rather than the rule. Many consultants felt that endoscopy was rather 'low brow' and not intellectually very challenging and were thus quite happy to delegate the responsibility to their junior staff. This was sadly very much the 'see one, do one, teach one' era of endoscopy.

In those early days, the teaching of not only endoscopic skills, but also sedation technique was incredibly patchy and poor. Patients who had their endoscopic procedure carried out in main theatre under either a general anaesthetic or intravenous sedation did in many ways best since in either case it would be an experienced anaesthetist who administered the sedative drugs and monitored the patient's vital signs.

In the 1970s in the UK, a patient undergoing a gastrointestinal endoscopic procedure would probably be sedated with intravenous diazepam with or without an opioid such as pethidine (Bell, 1990), the dosages employed often being much higher than are used today. When I was appointed a consultant in the department of therapeutics in Nottingham in 1976, I would have said that the most common fatal complications of upper gastrointestinal endoscopy were unquestionably haemorrhage and perforation, but we now know that this is totally incorrect since cardiopulmonary complications account for over half of the fatal complications of OGD. This message has sadly taken a long time to be heeded in some quarters.

In 1983 I moved from an academic unit at a teaching hospital with a well-established endoscopy unit to Ipswich Hospital in Suffolk. Here things were very different. Whereas 'surgical endoscopies' were performed in the main theatre under the watchful eye of an anaesthetist, 'medical endoscopies' were carried out just once a week in the sister's office of my predecessor's medical ward! After many battles, I managed to persuade the hospital to appoint its first endoscopy nurse, Anne Morden, who remained as sister-in-charge until her retirement in 1999. I was also lucky to have the help and support of my two surgical colleagues, Humphrey Adair and Ian Scott, during the setting up of the early unit. We moved a total of five times: from ward to outpatient department, from outpatients to ward, from ward to day theatre, from day theatre to ward and finally from ward to purpose-built endoscopy unit.

Soon after setting up the embryonic endoscopy unit at Ipswich, I decided to change from using intravenous diazepam to sedate my patients, to using the then recently released benzodiazepine midazolam. The manufacturer's literature suggested that midazolam was approximately twice as potent as diazepam and had the advantage of being water soluble, with a much shorter half-life. Within the first few weeks of using intravenous midazolam, I had several very frightening 'near misses' in terms of respiratory depression and one almost fatal respiratory arrest. In contrast, during my 7 years in Nottingham, I had had only one similar episode with intravenous diazepam despite carrying out several thousand upper gastrointestinal endoscopies. Midazolam was quite clearly considerably more than twice as potent as diazepam. We now know that midazolam is in fact probably 4–6 times stronger than diazepam.

Anne Morden and I were left with the choice of abandoning midazolam and going back to using diazepam (which appeared to be the safer option) or sticking with midazolam but being much more careful about its dosage. We decided on the latter, and for my next 800 cases, I or my registrar (first Gavin Spickett and then Paul Reeve) carefully titrated the intravenous midazolam over several minutes prior to carrying out the OGD (Bell et al., 1987a), the exact dose of midazolam being carefully recorded for later analysis. It soon became clear that older patients required a fraction of the dose of fit young people (Bell et al., 1987a). Intravenous midazolam was available only in a 10 mg/2 ml ampoule, so anybody simply giving an ampoule of the drug could potentially be giving over five times the dose necessary to sedate a frail 80-year-old. At that time, pulse oximeters were not available to monitor oxygen saturation, and the specific benzodiazepine antagonist flumazenil was not on general release, so it was hardly surprising that patients were getting into trouble.

We were very fortunate to have in Ipswich at that time an excellent and highly innovative respiratory physiologist by the name of Tom Coady, and as luck would have it, the respiratory physiology laboratory was very close to the day unit that was temporarily housing the endoscopy unit. I discussed with Tom the fact that we had had a number of life-threatening episodes of respiratory depression following the use of intravenous midazolam, and he very kindly allowed us to use his state-of-the-art ear oximeter to measure the oxygen saturation of the patients undergoing OGD. Equally importantly, he also lent us his very obliging chief technician, John Lee, a friend of Anne Morden's, on a regular basis for several years while we completed our research.

Our work confirmed that patients undergoing OGD under intravenous sedation often showed a marked fall in oxygen saturation as a result of drug-induced respiratory depression (Bell et al., 1987b). By using an induction plethysmograph vest calibrated using a pneumotachygraph, we could estimate respiratory tidal volume and minute volume. We were also able to show that the presence of an endoscope could compound the problem by producing a partial obstruction of the upper airways in a manner analogous to that seen in sleep apnoea: the greater the diameter of the gastroscope, the greater its propensity to cause hypoxia (Bell et al., 1987b). In addition, the combination of the ear oximeter, plethysmograph vest and calibrating pneumotachygraph allowed us to compare diazepam with midazolam in terms of drug-induced hypoxia (Bell et al., 1988) as well as study its reversal by the recently released antagonist flumazenil (Carter et al., 1990).

This work – and subsequent work on supplemental oxygen (Bell et al., 1987c), breathing patterns during OGD (Bell et al., 1991a, 1992), the comparison of winged needles versus plastic intravenous cannulae (Smith et al., 1993a) and the effect of a small bolus injection as opposed to the slow titration of benzodiazepines (Bell et al., 1990; Smith et al., 1993b) – would not have been possible without the help of successive registrars from the anaesthetic department at Ipswich Hospital who were lent to me for 6 month periods to give them research experience. I am indebted to the two consultant anaesthetic tutors, Don Elliot and Tony Nicholl, as well as the registrars themselves: Anna Carter, Hugh Antrobus, Maggie Smith and Barbara Fullerton.

One of my proudest moments was to speak with Harold Hopkin over the telephone after I was awarded the 1989 Hopkin's Endoscopy Prize on behalf of the Ipswich Hospital endoscopy unit for our work on sedation and monitoring. Professor Hopkin conceded that a successful endoscopic procedure was not much help to the patient if he or she then died as a result of the sedation!

In those early days, before research workers had their own computers with a nice statistical software package, I had to rely on outside help. Richard Logan, an epidemiologist/gastroenterologist at Nottingham, came to my aid with the initial analysis of the data relating the dose of midazolam to age and sex (Bell et al., 1987b). Richard also came up with the idea of sending out a questionnaire to all members of the BSG on current sedation practice. The questionnaire, which included a few questions relating to deaths and drug-induced cardiopulmonary complications following intravenous sedation, was analysed by Tawfique Daneshmend, lecturer in medicine on the therapeutics unit at Nottingham (Daneshmend et al., 1991). The results were startling, as were the results of a somewhat similar questionnaire study carried out in the USA (Arrowsmith et al., 1991). Our colleagues on the other side of the Atlantic were also waking up to the fact that the dose of midazolam used was too high – in fact at least 180 deaths in the USA were probably caused by this problem.

Christopher Williams, vice president and chairman of the influential Endoscopy Committee of the BSG, asked me whether I would chair a Working Party on the question of sedation and monitoring during gastrointestinal endoscopy and try to come up with some 'sensible suggestions'. I put together a group consisting of an endoscopy nurse

(Diane Campbell), an anaesthetist (Ed Charlton), two surgeon endoscopists (Rory McCloy and Mike Gear), a public health specialist (Neil Dent), an epidemiologist/gastroenterologist (Richard Logan) and myself, a gastroenterologist/general physician.

Opinion on the question of sedation and monitoring ranged from that of the 'flat earth brigade', who felt that no change was required, to that of the most hawkish, who felt that all sedation should be administered by an anaesthetist with full monitoring, including ECG, vital signs, pulse oximetry and end-tidal carbon dioxide monitoring. The document we produced, *Recommendations for standards of sedation and patient monitoring during gastrointestinal endoscopy* was severely criticised by both the Endoscopy Committee and the Council of the BSG. The final version, published in the journal *Gut* in 1991 was somewhat 'watered down' from the original document (Bell et al., 1991b). I like to think that our recommendations were reasonably sensible and helpful. The main recommendations were as follows:

1. Safety and monitoring should be part of a quality assurance programme for endoscopy units.
2. Resuscitation equipment and drugs must be available in the endoscopy and recovery areas.
3. Staff of all grades and disciplines should be familiar with resuscitation methods and undergo periodic retraining.
4. Equipment and drugs necessary for the maintenance of airway, breathing and circulation should be present in the endoscopy unit and recovery area (if outside the unit) and checked regularly.
5. A qualified nurse, trained in endoscopic techniques and adequately trained in resuscitation, should monitor the patient's condition during procedures.
6. Before endoscopy, adverse risk factors should be identified; this may be aided by the use of a check list.
7. The dosage of all drugs should be kept to the minimum necessary. There is evidence that benzodiazepine/opioid mixtures are hazardous.
8. Specific antagonists for benzodiazepines and opioids exist and should be available in the event of an emergency.
9. A cannula should be placed in a vein during the endoscopy of 'at-risk' patients.
10. Oxygen-enriched air should be given to 'at-risk' patients undergoing endoscopic procedures.

11. The endoscopist should ensure the well-being and clinical observation of the patient undergoing endoscopy in conjunction with another individual. This individual should be a qualified nurse trained in endoscopic techniques or another medically qualified practitioner.
12. Monitoring techniques such as pulse oximetry are recommended.
13. The clinical monitoring of the patient must continue into the recovery area.
14. Records of management and outcome should be collected and will provide data for appropriate audit.

Prospective audit of upper gastrointestinal endoscopy in two regions of England

At the time that the sedation standards document (Bell et al., 1991b) was published, there were plenty of endoscopists who felt that the working party's recommendations were 'totally over the top'. Some stated publicly that they *never* had any complications from their sedation technique and saw no need to reduce the dose of sedation, use an indwelling cannula, ever use oxygen or employ a pulse oximeter. The debate was useful in that it spawned a recommendation from the BSG Council that there should be a prospective audit of the whole question of safety, staffing and sedation methods. In view of the relative rarity of life-threatening cardiopulmonary adverse events, it was decided that the audit population would need to be very large. It was also decided that, in order to detect all adverse events (including, for example, aspiration pneumonia), it would be necessary to look at 30 day mortality/morbidity rather than simply the obvious cardiac arrests, episodes of respiratory depression and so on that occurred during or immediately after the endoscopic procedure.

The expert on postoperative 30 day mortality at the time was the late Brendan Devlin, a consultant surgeon who ran the Royal College of Surgeons (RCS) Confidential Enquiry into Perioperative Death (CEPOD) office in London. Brendan needed little persuasion to help us with the study. The BSG involved the RCS in London (Brendan Devlin), the Royal College of Physicians (RCP) Audit Department (Anthony Hopkin) and the Royal College of Anaesthetists (Ed Charlton) in the study. It was recognized that a large percentage of endoscopic procedures were being carried out by surgeons and GP clinical assistants, many of whom were not members of the BSG. It was therefore critically important to involve not only the RCS, but also the Association of Surgeons of Great Britain and Ireland and the Thoracic Society of Great Britain.

The two health regions chosen for the audit of upper gastrointestinal endoscopy were the North West (coordinated by Rory McCloy) and East Anglia (coordinated by myself). A full-time research fellow (Amanda Quine) was appointed for 2 years to run the study (Quine et al., 1995a). The ambitious aim was to try to include all the NHS units performing flexible diagnostic and therapeutic upper gastrointestinal endoscopy in the two regions. Amanda had the thankless task of visiting all units, endoscopists and endoscopy assistants throughout the North West and East Anglia. For a 4 month period, forms were completed by the endoscopists after each and every gastroscopy, these detailing where the procedure was performed, the experience of the endoscopist, the reason for the endoscopy, the nursing level, the sedation and monitoring details, and the outcome. When the procedures had been performed, the patient's notes were flagged requesting that any subsequent adverse event be reported to the endoscopy sister, who acted as a coordinator for the project at each site. Similarly, letters explaining the purpose of the audit were filed in the patients' notes and sent to the patients' GPs. All records relating to particular hospitals and particular doctors taking part in the study were coded so that it would not be possible to trace any adverse outcome to an individual hospital or doctor (Quine et al., 1995a).

Amanda contacted each unit on a 3-weekly basis to enquire about any problems with the audit, including the completion of the forms. The data were validated at the end of the study. Seven per cent of the completed forms were checked against the information in the hospital notes, showing a 95% accuracy rate in form completion. In addition, the total number of endoscopies performed by each unit was compared with the audit's total: compliance with the study was 99.9% on the endoscopy units, whereas in theatres the comparative figure was only 84.6% (Quine et al., 1995a). Any nurse reading this book who wishes to have full details of the forms used and the methods and validation process employed can contact the BSG Audit Office.

It was greatly to the credit of Amanda Quine that she managed to persuade 36 of the 39 hospitals in the two regions to take part in the study. As Amanda will admit, however, she was greatly helped by Brendan Devlin, who made it very clear to any reluctant individual surgeon that he or she had to have a very good reason not to participate. A total of 383 doctors, including 148 consultants, took part (Quine et al., 1995a). It was of interest that only 34% of the consultants taking part were members of the BSG – hence the importance of involving the RCS and RCP, and of the 'Devlin factor'. In the 4 month period from February to June 1991,

East Anglia performed 3956 upper gastrointestinal endoscopies (an estimated 5.76 gastroscopies per 1000 general population per year), the North West carrying out 10 193 examinations (8.8 per 1000 population per year) in the 4 month period April–August 1991. The total number of procedures performed was 14 149, of which 13 036 (92%) were diagnostic and the rest therapeutic. Thirty per cent of patients were over the age of 70 years. Only half of the patients were categorized as ASA grade I (in the American Society of Anesthesiologists' classification of physical status), whereas over 10% of the patients fell into grades III–V (i.e. high-risk groups). In East Anglia and the North West at that time, 21% and 25% of examinations respectively were conducted either with only one nurse in attendance or with two unqualified nurses (Quine et al., 1995a).

In East Anglia and the North West, 4.4% and 2.3% respectively of all gastroscopies were performed under a general anaesthetic. The figures for procedures taking place without sedation or local anaesthesia, with local anaesthetic alone and with some form of intravenous sedation (with or without local anaesthetic), were 2.3% and 0.4%, 7.1% and 12.6%, and 86% and 84% respectively. The mean doses of diazepam used for sedation in the two regions were 13.5mg and 14.0mg respectively, whereas that for midazolam was 5.7mg in both regions. The distribution of dosages used was very wide, so that a consideration of mean doses used was unhelpful on its own without reference to age or ASA grouping. The maximum dose of diazepam and midazolam used was 50mg and 30mg respectively, and although the mean dosage fell with advancing age, many frail elderly patients received dosages of sedation that were, in my view, frankly dangerous. One would have predicted that if an opioid such as pethidine were used in combination with diazepam or midazolam for a diagnostic examination, the dose of the benzodiazepine would have been lower than if it were used as the sole intravenous sedative agent, but in fact the reverse was true in practice: with the average dose of 50mg pethidine, the mean dose of diazepam or midazolam was actually *higher* than was seen when using the benzodiazepine alone (Quine et al., 1995a).

The two regions differed markedly in their use of the recently introduced intravenous benzodiazepine antagonist flumazenil. Whereas 428 patients (4.2%) in the North West were given intravenous flumazenil, the corresponding figure for East Anglia was just 20 (0.5%). Twenty-two per cent of the doses in East Anglia, but only 3.6% of those in the North West, were employed in an emergency to reverse benzodiazepine-induced respiratory depression. Thus, much of the non-urgent use of flumazenil in the North West was to reverse residual sedation when adequate staffing levels and recovery areas could not be provided (Quine et al., 1995a). Endoscopists also differed widely in their use of continuous intravenous access, pulse oximetry and supplementary oxygen (Quine et al., 1995a). Overall, cannulae were used in 12.8% of cases and 'butterflies' (winged steel needles) in 30%; 40% of patients were endoscoped with the aid of pulse oximetry, and only 12.5% were given oxygen supplementation throughout. Of particular concern were the figures relating to ASA grades III–V, the 'high-risk groups': only 15% of these (sedated) in the North West were given oxygen during the procedure, and only 37% had continuous intravenous access.

This study was the first large, prospective audit of endoscopy-related deaths and complications, and included events occurring up to 30 days after upper gastrointestinal endoscopy in over 14 000 patients. A variety of complications were reported to the local co-ordinators (see Quine et al., 1995a, 1995b); in summary, 104 patients died within the 30 day period of follow-up, and in at least seven cases, these deaths were related to the procedure, thus giving, at even a conservative estimate, a death rate of 1 in 2000. When one bears in mind that anaesthetic-related deaths following a general anaesthetic occur with only about 1 in 100 000 operations, this shows just how appalling the endoscopy figures really were.

Other complications might have been related to the performance of the procedure. There were 11 cases of pneumonia, 6 cerebrovascular accidents and 19 myocardial infarctions, 24 out of 36 (67%) of these complications occurring within 7 days of the procedure. There were also plenty of 'near misses', including five cardiac arrests either during or shortly after the procedure. All the patients were initially successfully resuscitated, but one died 4 days later from an aspiration pneumonia. Cardiopulmonary complications were reported in 31 cases, many of which required flumazenil and oxygen therapy. Despite the fact that some of these patients were ASA grades II–IV, intravenous access and pulse oximetry were not invariably used, and supplemental oxygen appeared to be the exception rather than the rule (Quine et al., 1995a).

At the time of this study, only 11% of OGDs were performed with just local anaesthetic spray: if the same audit were carried out today, the figure would be much higher. It should be remembered that lignocaine is a respiratory depressant and can also cause hypotension, bradycardia and cardiac arrest, and that these effects can be potentiated by benzodiazepines. Pharyngeal anaesthesia, combined with the presence of the gastroscope, which interferes with glottic closure and swallowing, is known to predispose to pulmonary aspiration; 10 out of 11 of the patients reported in the audit to have developed pneumonia shortly after the procedure had received local anaesthesia. It was a sobering finding that 8 of these 11 patients died (Quine et al., 1995a). Only two of these cases were adjudged to have resulted directly from the procedure as the episode of aspiration was recorded on the unit immediately after or during the procedure, but there was a suspicion that several (if not all) of the other cases were also procedure related. If one needs to gastroscope a patient at high risk of aspiration, for example someone with gastric outlet obstruction or a large gastrointestinal haemorrhage, it is probably safer to use either intravenous sedation or local anaesthetic alone – but not both (Quine et al., 1995a).

The doses of benzodiazepine actually given could be at least double the manufacturer's recommended dose range, particularly serious being the dosage sometimes employed for frail elderly patients. Take as an example an 83-year-old man of ASA grade III who developed a cerebrovascular accident immediately after the gastroscopy and died 7 days later. The dose of midazolam used (4mg) almost certainly caused both hypotension and hypoxia, thus precipitating his cerebrovascular accident. The patient did not have an indwelling cannula, an oximeter or the benefit of supplemental oxygen. I never use more than 2mg intravenous midazolam in anyone over the age of 70 years; for an 83-year-old, I would use a maximum of 1.0–1.5mg of the drug.

The BSG had recommended that endoscopies should ideally be performed in well-designed units, yet in this study over 25% of the procedures were still being carried out at other sites. Even 8 years after the audit, many endoscopists still work on endoscopy units that are converted wards, day units or day theatres, where the staff are plagued by many problems – poor access, poor waiting areas and poor or non-existent storage space for equipment. Particularly memorable were a couple of the units in the North West region, which were housed in small rooms previously disused, situated off a distant corridor with no recovery area whatsoever. The BSG also recommends that two assistants, at least one of whom must be a qualified nurse (RGN or EN), are required at each table, yet in 3 of the 36 hospitals that participated in the audit (Quine et al., 1995a), entire lists were being carried out with just a single unqualified nurse.

Royal College of Surgeons guidelines for sedation by non-anaesthetists

The RCS Working Party on sedation by non-anaesthetists met in 1992 and published its recommendations in 1993. Although the 'Quine report' (Quine et al., 1995a) was not finally published until 1995, the results were known to members of the RCS working party. Based on the alarmingly high morbidity and mortality figures in the 1991 audit, the Working Party was able to make rather stronger recommendations (McCloy et al., 1993) than the original BSG Working Party (Bell et al., 1991b). In particular, it recommended that *all* patients (rather than just 'at-risk' patients) undergoing endoscopic procedures under intravenous sedation should have continuous venous access during both the procedure itself and the early recovery stage, monitoring by pulse oximetry, and supplemental oxygen. In addition, much firmer advice could be given regarding choice of benzodiazepine (midazolam being preferred) and a more sensible dosage, particularly for elderly people.[1]

One of the most controversial recommendations has been the use of supplemental oxygen for all patients, as opposed to only 'at-risk' patients, undergoing procedures under sedation. I have repeatedly argued the case for routine supplemental oxygen (Bell, 1992; Smith and Bell, 1994; Bell and Jones, 1996). The question of whether the ST segment changes seen during continuous ECG monitoring in some patients are caused mainly by tachycardia or by hypoxia has been reviewed at length (Lazzaroni and Bianco-Porro, 1999) – it is probably a combination of both. Any cardiologist wishing to look for evidence of myocardial ischaemia will order a treadmill stress test rather than get the patient to inhale a hypoxic gas mixture. An anaesthetist will try to keep myocardial oxygen demand down by avoiding stress, significant tachycardia and dangerous rises in blood pressure. At the same time, he or she will try to optimize myocardial oxygen supply by avoiding bradycardia or hypotension, ensuring an adequate haemoglobin concentration and, finally, preventing hypoxia by appropriately ventilating the patient with oxygen-enriched air (Bell and Jones, 1996).

The subject of hypoxaemia at the time of gastroscopy, colonoscopy or ERCP has been reviewed on numerous occasions (Bell, 1990, 1992, 2000,

[1] Since the preparation of this chapter, the Academy of Medical Royal Colleges (AOMRC) has published a further Report of an Intercollegiate Working Party chaired by the Royal College of Anaesthetists (November, 2001), entitled *Implementing and Ensuring Safe Sedation Practice for Healthcare Procedures in Adults* (see Chapter 8).

2002; Smith and Bell, 1994; Bell and Jones, 1996; Whitwam and McCloy, 1998; Freeman, 1999; Lazzaroni and Bianco-Porro, 1999). It is considered unacceptable in anaesthetic circles for the oxygen saturation level to fall below 85% (Charlton, 1995), yet authors still blithely report falls of this magnitude (Wehrmann et al., 1999; Reimann et al., 2000). Such levels are frankly dangerous, and the routine use of supplemental oxygen would have greatly reduced this unnecessary risk to patients (Bell, 1992; Smith and Bell, 1994; Charlton, 1995; Bell and Jones, 1996; Bell, 2000).

References

Arrowsmith J, Gerstman B, Fleischer D, Benjamin S (1991) Results from the American Society for Gastrointestinal Endoscopy/US Food and Drug Administration collaborative study on complication rates and drug use during gastrointestinal endoscopy. Gastrointestinal Endoscopy 37: 421–7.

Bell GD (1990) Premedication and IV sedation for upper gastrointestinal endoscopy. Alimentary Pharmacology and Therapeutics 4: 103–22.

Bell GD (1992) Who is for supplemental oxygen? Gastrointestinal Endoscopy 38: 514–16 (editorial).

Bell GD (2000) Premedication, preparation, and surveillance. In: State of the Art in Gastroenterologic Endoscopy – A Review of Last Year's Most Significant Publications. Endoscopy 32: 92–100.

Bell GD (2002) Premedication, preparation, and surveillance. In: State of the Art in Gastroenterologic Endoscopy – A Review of Last Year's Most Significant Publications. Endoscopy 34: 1–11.

Bell GD, Jones JG (1996) Routine use of pulse oximetry and supplemental oxygen during endoscopic procedures under conscious sedation: British beef or common sense? Endoscopy 28: 718–21 (editorial).

Bell GD, Spickett GP, Reeve P, Morden A, Logan RFA (1987a) Intravenous midazolam for upper gastrointestinal endoscopy: a study of 800 consecutive cases relating dose to age and sex of patient. British Journal of Clinical Pharmacology 23: 241–3.

Bell GD, Reeve P, Moshiri M et al. (1987b) Intravenous midazolam: a study of the degree of oxygen desaturation occurring during upper gastrointestinal endoscopy. British Journal of Clinical Pharmacology 23: 703–708.

Bell GD, Bown NS, Morden A, Coady T, Logan RFA (1987c) Prevention of hypoxaemia during upper gastrointestinal endoscopy using supplemental oxygen via nasal cannulae. Lancet i: 1022–3.

Bell GD, Morden A, Coady T, Lee J, Logan RFA (1988) A comparison of diazepam and midazolam as endoscopy premedication assessing changes in ventilation and oxygen desaturation. British Journal of Clinical Pharmacology 26: 595–600.

Bell GD, Antrobus JHL, Lee J, Coady T, Morden A (1990) Bolus or slow titrated injection of midazolam prior to OGD? Relative effect on oxygen saturation and prophylactic value of supplemental oxygen. Alimentary Pharmacology and Therapeutics 4: 393–401.

Bell GD, Antrobus JHL, Lee J, Coady T, Morden A (1991a) Pattern of breathing during upper gastrointestinal endoscopy – implications for administration of supplemental oxygen. Alimentary Pharmacology and Therapeutics 5: 399–404.

Bell GD, McCloy RF, Charlton JE et al. (1991b) Recommendations for standards of sedation and patient monitoring during gastrointestinal endoscopy. Gut 32: 823–7.

Bell GD, Quine A, Antrobus JHL et al. (1992) Upper gastrointestinal endoscopy: a prospective randomized study comparing the efficacy of continuous supplemental oxygen given either via the nasal or oral route. Gastrointestinal Endoscopy 38: 319–25.

Carter A, Bell GD, Coady T, Lee J, Morden A (1990) Speed of reversal of midazolam-induced respiratory depression by flumazenil following gastroscopy. Acta Anaesthesiologica Scandinavica 34 (Suppl 92): 59–64.

Charlton JE (1995) Monitoring and supplemental oxygen during endoscopy. British Medical Journal 310: 886–7 (editorial).

Daneshmend TK, Bell GD, Logan RFA (1991) Sedation for upper gastrointestinal endoscopy: results of a nationwide survey. Gut 32: 12–15.

Freeman ML (1999) Sedation and monitoring for gastrointestinal endoscopy. In Yamada T, Alpers DH, Laine L, Owyang C, Powell DW (eds) Textbook of Gastroenterology, 3rd edn. Philadelphia: Lippincott Williams & Wilkins.

Lazzaroni M, Bianco-Porro G (1999) Premedication, preparation and surveillance. Endoscopy 31(1): 2–8.

Le Fanu J (1999) The Rise and Fall of Modern Medicine. London: Little, Brown.

McCloy RF, Bell GD, Skelly AM et al. (1993) Guidelines for Sedation by Non-Anaesthetists. Report of a Working Party of the Royal College of Surgeons. London: RCS.

Quine MA, Bell GD, McCloy RF, Charlton JE, Devlin HB, Hopkin A (1995a) Prospective audit of upper gastrointestinal endoscopy in two regions of England: safety, staffing and sedation methods. Gut 36: 462–7.

Quine MA, Bell GD, McCloy RF, Mathews HR (1995b) Prospective audit of perforation rates following upper gastrointestinal endoscopy in two regions in England. British Journal of Surgery 82: 530–3.

Reimann FM, Samson U, Derad I, Fuchs M, Schiefer B, Stange EF (2000) Synergistic sedation with low dose midazolam and propofol for colonoscopy. Endoscopy 32: 239–44.

Salmon PR (1974) Recent developments in gastrointestinal endoscopy. In: Truelove SC, Trowell J (Eds) Topics in Gastroenterology 2. Oxford: Blackwell Scientific Publications.

Smith M, Bell GD (1994) Routine oxygen during endoscopy. Endoscopy 21: 301–2 (editorial).

Smith M, Bell GD, Fullerton B, Quine S, Morden A (1993a) A comparison of winged steel needles and Teflon cannulas in maintaining intravenous access during gastrointestinal endoscopy. Gastrointestinal Endoscopy 39: 33–6.

Smith M, Bell GD, Quine A, Spencer GM, Morden A, Jones G (1993b) Small bolus injections of intravenous midazolam for upper gastrointestinal endoscopy: a study of 788 consecutive cases. British Journal of Clinical Pharmacology 36: 573–8.

Wehrmann T, Kokabpick S, Lembcke B, Caspary WF, Seifert H (1999) Efficacy and safety of intravenous propofol sedation during routine ERCP: a prospective, controlled study. Gastrointestinal Endoscopy 49: 677–83.

Whitwam JG, McCloy RF (1998) Principles and Practice of Sedation, 2nd edn. Oxford: Blackwell Scientific.

CHAPTER 2

Physiology and pharmacology of sedation agents

CAROLE BOYLE

The ideal drug used for sedation should be potent with a rapid onset of action, have no side effects and possess a short duration of action, thus allowing the patient to return to normal life immediately after treatment. There should be no prescribing restrictions, and the drug itself should be inexpensive.

Unfortunately, the ideal drug does not yet exist, and all the drugs available have some side effects and cause physiological changes. The drugs currently used are the benzodiazepines for intravenous sedation and nitrous oxide for inhalational sedation. The pharmacology of and physiological changes caused by these drugs will be discussed in this chapter. Other agents such as propofol and sevoflurane, although not as widely used, will also be covered.

Basic principles

Drugs that produce conscious sedation and/or analgesia can be administered by a variety of methods: oral, inhalational, rectal and via injection, either intravenous or intramuscular. Other methods include sublingual and intranasal administration, although currently these routes are not often used in the UK to provide conscious sedation. The choice of route depends on the drug itself, how quickly a response is required and whether the effect is required locally or systemically.

Oral administration is more pleasant for a patient who is scared of needles, but absorption into the bloodstream from the stomach and gastrointestinal tract will be slow. The rate of gastric emptying is important in determining the rate of absorption and is altered by disease, other drugs and the presence of food. Drugs are also subject to first-pass metabolism as the portal veins drain blood to the liver, where metabolism takes place before the agent can reach its receptor site and be effective.

Drugs administered by inhalation are absorbed via the pulmonary circulation. This route is useful for drugs that act directly on the lung tissue, for example those found in the inhalers used in asthma, and drugs that act centrally, such as anaesthetic gases.

Parenteral (by injection) administration is, in contrast, much faster acting; drugs used in an emergency are almost all given by this method. This route does, however, have some disadvantages, for example allergic reactions will occur much more quickly to an intravenously administered drug than to the same drug administered orally.

Pharmacokinetics

'Pharmacokinetics' describes the effect that the patient has on the drug, relating to the way in which the drug is absorbed, distributed round the body, metabolized and finally excreted.

The degree of protein binding determines the effectiveness of the drug. When a drug has been absorbed, it travels to its target receptors in the plasma. Some of the drug – the active part – is dissolved in the plasma, the rest being bound to plasma proteins and therefore inactive. The amount of protein binding can vary in patients who are unwell, for example those with renal or hepatic disease, as they may have a reduced level of plasma proteins. Two drugs can compete for the same binding site and thereby increase the free concentration of one or both agents. This competition is not clinically significant for sedative agents but can be for other drugs. Aspirin, for example, displaces warfarin from its binding sites and can lead to excessive bleeding.

Drugs are eliminated by a variety of routes. The most important organs are the liver and kidneys, via which most drugs are metabolized and excreted. Inhalational agents are excreted through the lungs. The measure of elimination of the drug is the half-life, which is the time taken to reduce the amount of drug available in the plasma to half the original dose.

The pharmacokinetics of a drug has clinical significance. With agents used for sedation, a fast absorption and distribution mean that the patient will not have to wait long for the sedative effect. If a drug undergoes rapid metabolism and excretion, there will be a swift recovery and faster discharge for the patient.

Pharmacodynamics

Pharmacodynamics relates to the effect that the drug has on the patient, considering both the desirable and the undesirable effects. Most, although not all, drugs elicit a response via receptors that are specific for each drug, these receptors being found in the cell membranes. If a drug binds to a receptor, the receptor is altered and the cell is stimulated to produce a result that can be measured; such drugs are called agonists. Drugs that compete for the same receptor sites and therefore block the action of agonists are known as antagonists. A third type of drug that binds to the receptor site is the inverse agonist; this drug produces the opposite effect to the agonist. A benzodiazepine inverse agonist will, for example, produce anxiety rather than sedation. Antagonists will also compete with inverse agonists for receptor sites.

Benzodiazepines

The first benzodiazepine, chlordiazepoxide (Librium), was synthesized in 1955 at Hoffman La Roche, diazepam (Valium) entering clinical practice in 1963. Midazolam (Hypnovel) was discovered later and became available in the UK in 1983 for intravenous sedation. Its advantages over diazepam have made it the drug of choice for intravenous sedation. Other benzodiazepines include temazepam, which is used for oral sedation, and lorazepam.

The benzodiazepines have a number of properties that make them useful for sedation: they produce anxiolysis, muscle relaxation, hypnosis and amnesia. The drugs have a common core structure but differences that determine their solubility and precise action.

Diazepam

Diazepam produces excellent sedation but has a number of disadvantages. It is insoluble in water, and the first commercially available preparation, Valium, contained 5mg/ml of the drug in organic solvents including propylene glycol, ethyl alcohol and sodium benzoate in benzoic acid. The intravenous injection of Valium can be painful and can cause thrombophlebitis even as late as 7–10 days after injection. In another preparation, Diazemuls, the diazepam is dissolved in soya bean oil, which is non-irritant and does not damage the veins.

Midazolam

Midazolam (Figure 2.1) was first introduced as 10mg of drug in 2ml ampoules. It is stable in aqueous solution and non-irritant on injection. It is at least 2–3 times as potent as diazepam, and the initial preparation led to problems of oversedation as it was difficult to administer 2ml in small increments. Midazolam was subsequently produced as 10mg in 5ml, which is easier to titrate, 'titration' meaning giving the drug slowly in very small amounts while watching the patient's response. This method of administration is different from that of anaesthetic drugs, which are given on a dose per weight basis.

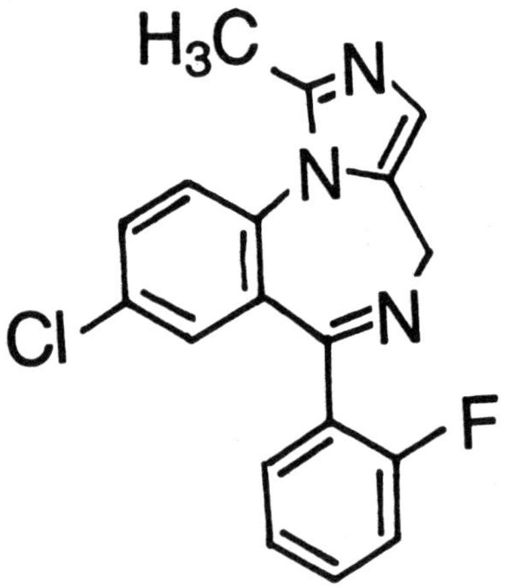

Figure 2.1 The structure of midazolam

In the UK, midazolam is only produced in a form suitable for intravenous administration, but this formulation has been mixed with other liquids to be administered orally and has also, in the 2ml formulation, been used intranasally. These methods of administration are useful for patients who cannot accept intravenous injections.

Temazepam

Temazepam is a minor metabolite of diazepam that is impossible to prepare as a solution; it is therefore not available for intravenous administration. Temazepam has been produced in various forms: tablet, gel-filled capsule and elixir for oral administration. The capsule formulation has, however, been withdrawn because of inappropriate intravenous use by drug users, particularly in the west of Scotland. It is now a Schedule 3 Controlled Drug and must be stored in a locked cupboard. Temazepam is currently not as strictly regulated as the Schedule 2 drugs such as morphine, which must be logged in a register signed by the members of staff administering the drug.

The different formulations have different rates of absorption, but temazepam is generally rapidly absorbed following oral administration, the sedative effects usually being clinically apparent after 45–60 minutes. Temazepam has a short half-life of 5–11 hours, which makes it a useful drug for sedation and for premedication before general anaesthesia.

Flumazenil

Flumazenil (Anexate; Figure 2.2) is a specific benzodiazepine antagonist. It has the same core structure as the other benzodiazepines, which means that a patient who exhibits an allergic reaction to another benzodiazepine is highly likely to have an allergy to flumazenil. It has a stronger affinity for the benzodiazepine receptor than do the other benzodiazepines and will therefore displace them. Flumazenil itself has no clinically apparent sedative or stimulant effects on the CNS but will reverse previous sedation and cause the patient to awaken.

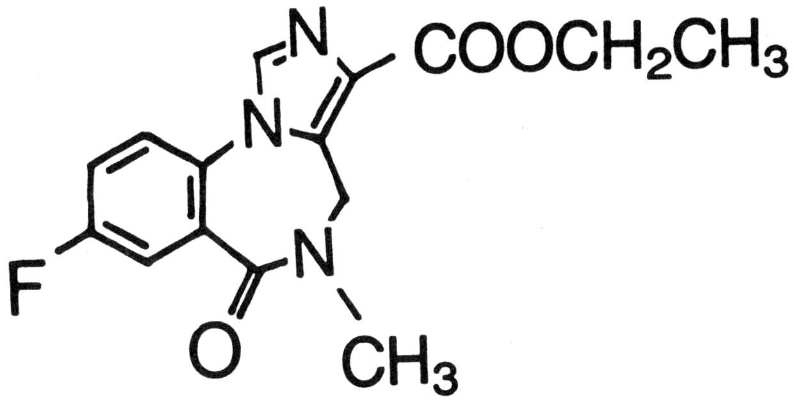

Figure 2.2 The structure of flumazenil

Flumazenil has a shorter half-life than midazolam, and when it was first introduced in 1988 there was a suggestion that sedated patients would become re-sedated 50–60 minutes after reversal because of the remaining midazolam. The displaced benzodiazepine continues, however, to be distributed and metabolized at the normal rate, so after the effectiveness of flumazenil has worn off, the plasma level of midazolam is unlikely to be high enough to cause sedation. Re-sedation is not a problem following a single dose but may cause difficulties if continuous infusions or repeated doses of benzodiazepine are being used for sedation, for example in intensive care.

Pharmacodynamics

The benzodiazepines act on specific receptors in the CNS and at other sites throughout the body, including the myocardium. Benzodiazepine receptors are always closely associated with gamma-aminobutyric acid (GABA-A) receptors on neuronal cell membranes. GABA is an important inhibitory neurotransmitter in the brain, the physiological effect of GABA system inhibition being to dampen or filter out unnecessary sensory information. This maintains a balance between what is necessary for survival and normal functioning, and an overload of sensory stimuli.

The benzodiazepines have two actions at the receptors: first, facilitating the inhibitory actions of GABA, and second, mimicking the inhibitory action of glycine, which is the major neurotransmitter in the spinal cord and brainstem. These actions at receptor level are responsible for the clinical effects of the benzodiazepines. Sedation and anticonvulsant activity are caused by an increase in GABA transmission across the cell membranes. Copying the effect of glycine causes muscle relaxation and reduces anxiety. This indirect mode of action explains the high safety ratio of the benzodiazepines as their actions are limited to the maximal response to GABA.

The unusual effects exhibited in some patients who have been sedated using benzodiazepines can be explained by events at the receptor level. Patients who are, or have been, drug users may have an altered neurotransmitter profile and be difficult to sedate, instead becoming hyperactive and agitated. The elderly, who have a reduced number of receptors and a slower circulation time, are very sensitive to the effects of benzodiazepines and require sedative drugs to be given slowly and usually in much smaller doses.

The speed of onset and duration of action of the different benzodiazepines depend on their effect on the receptors. Midazolam and diazepam have a greater affinity for the benzodiazepine receptor than does lorazepam, which means that they have a rapid onset of action, making them suitable sedative drugs for outpatient procedures. Conversely, diazepam and midazolam dissociate from the receptor more quickly than temazepam, which makes temazepam a more suitable drug for night sedation.

Pharmacokinetics

The benzodiazepines have to cross the blood–brain barrier to reach their target receptors. This is a passive diffusion process, the rate of which depends on lipid solubility and protein binding. The different agents vary in their lipid solubility, although all are lipophilic; after a single intravenous injection, they rapidly cross the blood–brain barrier. Highly soluble agents such as diazepam and midazolam reach receptors in the brain more quickly than does the less soluble chlordiazepoxide.

All the benzodiazepines are bound to plasma albumin, although the degree of binding varies between different agents. Patients who have hypoalbuminaemia as a result of liver or kidney disease will show an enhanced clinical effect and should be sedated very carefully. No other drugs appear to compete with the benzodiazepines for binding sites on the plasma proteins.

After intravenous injection, the agents are distributed to the organs that receive the greatest blood supply: the CNS, heart, liver and kidneys. From these organs, the benzodiazepines are distributed to muscle and then to fat stores. This is significant in obese patients, who can store a large amount of benzodiazepine and take longer to recover from sedation.

Metabolism takes place in the liver and is measured by the clearance half-life. Different benzodiazepines have different biotransformation pathways, and some of their metabolites have a longer elimination half-life than the original agent. This occurs with diazepam, whose metabolite desmethyl diazepam also has a sedative effect. This is partly responsible for the hangover effect that can follow sedation with diazepam. Midazolam has no long-acting active metabolites and possesses a faster clearance than diazepam, resulting in faster recovery.

The benzodiazepines are excreted via the kidneys. The majority of the drug is excreted in the form of metabolites, although some drug is excreted unchanged. The ratio of changed to unchanged drug varies between the different drugs, only 1% of midazolam being excreted unchanged. Flumazenil is extensively broken down in the liver and even less is excreted in the urine.

Physiological effects of the benzodiazepines

Central nervous system

The main effect of the benzodiazepines on the CNS is depression. This is dose related, the clinical effect varying between the different drugs from mild sedation to the induction of general anaesthesia. Other effects on the CNS include hypnosis, amnesia, muscle relaxation and anticonvulsant activity.

The anticonvulsant effect of the benzodiazepines has been recognized for some time, diazepam being the recommended drug to treat status epilepticus. Midazolam is also effective in controlling fits but is not licensed for use in this way. There is, however, some benefit in using midazolam electively for epileptic individuals, rather than treating them without sedation, in order to reduce the likelihood of anxiety-induced fits.

The amnesia produced by the benzodiazepines is anterograde, which means that patients will not remember events occurring after an injection has taken place, although they will remember what happens before the drug takes effect. The lack of memory of unpleasant surgical events is a definite advantage for most patients and can be the main reason for using sedation for some surgery. The amnesia will last approximately 20–30 minutes, but this varies between patients. It is better not to guarantee patients total amnesia as it has been shown that amnesia is not totally reliable, particularly at lower doses. As midazolam-induced amnesia may be considerably prolonged in some people, it is essential to warn patients and their escorts or carers of this possibility.

Muscle relaxation can be useful in people who have involuntary movements. In patients with Parkinson's disease, for example, sedation can reduce movement, making investigations and treatment possible. The effect may also be advantageous for some surgical procedures in which relaxation makes surgical access easier, but it contributes to the difficulty in standing experienced by many patients at the end of their treatment.

Respiratory system

The main effect of the benzodiazepines on the respiratory system is depression. This is usually mild and insignificant in normal healthy patients if the drug is administered intravenously by slow titration, but it can be significant in unwell or elderly people. Even in fit healthy patients, a fast bolus of a large amount of a benzodiazepine can stop respiration. There are two ways in which the benzodiazepines affect respiration, the first being by reducing the sensitivity of the carbon dioxide receptors that are found in the respiratory centre in the brainstem. An increase in blood level of carbon dioxide is usually followed by an increase in respiration, but this response does not occur as efficiently when benzodiazepines are present in the circulation. The second effect on respiration is caused by relaxation of the muscles of respiration, including the intercostal muscles and diaphragm.

It is therefore important to monitor respiration during sedation, especially with intravenous sedation but also after the oral administration of benzodiazepines. Respiration can be monitored clinically, and it is important to look at a patient's depth and rate of breathing. It is not always easy to detect small changes in respiration, so electronic monitoring with a pulse oximeter is mandatory with intravenous sedation. This technique has been in standard use for anaesthesia since the mid-1980s and provides a non-invasive way of continuously monitoring pulse and oxygen saturation.

The pulse oximeter consists of two parts, a box containing a microprocessor with a display, and a probe that attaches to a finger or earlobe. Inside the probe are two light-emitting diodes (LEDs) and a single photo detector. One LED is for red light, the other for infrared. The probe picks up the colour of the blood by comparing the absorption of the two different wavelengths of light by pulsatile blood. The colour of the blood in turn denotes the level of oxygen saturation of the haemoglobin. The probe gives a reading only of the oxygenation of the blood; it does not indicate the amount of haemoglobin present in the blood and will not detect anaemia. A small proportion of oxygen is carried in the blood dissolved in the plasma, but the amount is so small as to be clinically insignificant, and this oxygen is not detected by pulse oximetry. The LEDs are not influenced by skin colour and record only pulsatile blood, so venous blood is not monitored.

Pulse oximetry readings are given as a percentage saturation based on the oxygen–haemoglobin dissociation curve (Figure 2.3), a graph that plots the percentage oxygen saturation against the oxygen tension (partial pressure) in the blood. Arterial oxygen is almost 100% saturated and has a partial pressure of 13.3 kPa (100 mmHg), whereas venous blood is 70% saturated and has a partial pressure of 5.3 kPa (40 mmHg). The graph is not linear because of the way in which the oxygen molecules combine with the haemoglobin molecule, each molecule of haemoglobin combining loosely and reversibly with four molecules of oxygen. As the blood moves to the periphery, oxygen is transferred to the tissues. The first molecule of oxygen is difficult to remove from the haemoglobin – this relating to the flat part of the curve – but when this oxygen has been lost, it becomes easier to give up subsequent molecules – the second steeper part of the curve. At the upper end of the curve, a reduction in 2% oxygen saturation represents a fall in the partial pressure of oxygen of about 15% (see Chapter 5).

The normal value for oxygen saturation is approximately 97–100%, although older people, smokers and those with respiratory disease will

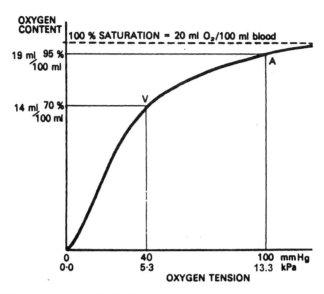

Figure 2.3 The oxygen–haemoglobin dissociation curve

demonstrate a lower value. During intravenous sedation, the low-saturation alarm will usually be set at 90% (just before the steeper part of the curve is reached). If the alarm sounds during treatment, the patient must first be assessed. The most common cause of the alarm sounding is detachment from the finger, so this should be checked and the probe replaced if necessary. If the saturation has dropped to below 90%, the patient should be asked to take some deep breaths as well-sedated patients often appear to forget to breathe. If this simple measure does not resolve the drop in oxygen saturation, positive-pressure oxygen and flumazenil will be required.

For individuals with compromised respiratory and/or cardiac function who have a low baseline oxygen saturation, oxygen can be administered throughout treatment via either an oxygen mask or nasal cannulae; the latter do not restrict access to the mouth. Oxygen, at a flow rate of 2–3 litres per minute, should be started before the administration of intravenous sedation and continued into the postoperative recovery period. It is important to be aware that pulse oximetry readings will be artificially high when the subject is breathing oxygen-enriched rather than room air.

Cardiovascular system

The cardiovascular effects of the benzodiazepines are slight and insignificant in healthy patients: there is a decrease in mean arterial pressure, cardiac output, stroke volume and systemic vascular resistance.

Clinically, this may present as a fall in blood pressure immediately after the intravenous injection of midazolam. This decrease in blood pressure is followed by a compensatory rise in heart rate, mediated by the baroreceptor reflex. Even in cardiovascularly compromised individuals, these cardiovascular effects are not usually a problem when a slow titration method is employed to produce sedation.

Propofol

Propofol is an anaesthetic induction agent that was introduced into clinical use in 1986, since when it has, because of its rapid onset of action, short duration and fast recovery time, become the agent of choice for day case surgery.

Propofol is an synthetic agent that is extremely lipid soluble but almost completely insoluble in water. The drug comes dissolved in a white, aqueous solution containing soya bean oil and purified egg phosphatide, each 20ml ampoule containing 200mg of propofol (10mg/ml). The solution is painful on injection, but this can be alleviated either by mixing it with lignocaine or by injecting a small dose of lignocaine (10mg) into the vein first. Using a larger vein also helps to reduce the pain.

The pharmacokinetic properties of propofol that make it an ideal agent for day case general anaesthesia also make it suitable, in lower doses, for sedation. Following an initial injection, propofol is distributed to the brain and peripheral tissues. The distribution half-life is 1.8–4.1 seconds. Clearance from the plasma is rapid, and it has been suggested that organs other than just the liver are involved in its metabolism. The metabolites of propofol are excreted by the kidneys, only 0.3% being excreted unchanged.

Propofol is useful for short procedures when sedation is required for only minutes as patients recover very quickly. It is also a good agent for long procedures, maybe lasting hours, as the elimination rate is not altered by long infusion times.

Opioids

For some patients, the use of a single agent does not provide the degree of sedation required, a combination of agents often providing better sedation conditions. The most frequently used agents are the opioids, which are more commonly used for systemic analgesia. The opioids, like the benzodiazepines, act through receptors and can have agonistic or antagonistic actions. The group has a number of effects in addition to analgesia, including respiratory depression, muscle rigidity, tolerance and nausea and vomiting. All of these effects are significant for sedation, but the most important is respiratory depression, and great care must be taken when a combination of opioid and benzodiazepine is used for sedation.

The drugs most frequently used in this way for sedation are nalbuphine and fentanyl or alfentanil. Nalbuphine has the advantage that it is not a controlled drug, so that, unlike the other opioids, special precautions are not required for its storage. It is usually given first in a fixed dose of 5–10mg, midazolam then being titrated to give a suitable level of sedation. The incidence of vomiting is high using this technique, and it may be necessary to administer an antiemetic postoperatively. Fentanyl and alfentanil are controlled drugs but are, especially alfentanil, shorter acting; they can be given in small doses before the administration of a benzodiazepine. If opioids are used for sedation, the opioid antagonist naloxone must be available. Naloxone is a pure antagonist for the opioids. As it will reverse both respiratory depression and analgesia, it is best given by titration in small increments rather than as a bolus dose if it is important to retain some analgesic effect.

Inhalational sedation agents

Inhalational agents are less commonly used for sedation because of the inconvenient equipment required and the need to administer the gas via a mask. Nitrous oxide has traditionally been the only gas used for sedation and analgesia, most notably in obstetrics, but other agents are now being used and may have a role to play in the future.

The most notable advantage of gaseous administration over intravenous administration is that venepuncture is not required, which may be better for both operator and patient. Inhaled drugs are taken into the lungs, rapid sedation following as a result of the large epithelial surface available for absorption. The rate of absorption depends on a number of factors, including the solubility of the drug in blood: an agent with a high solubility in blood will be rapidly taken up and the alveolar concentration, which reflects the brain concentration, will increase only slowly to the desired level. Conversely, a less-soluble agent will show a more rapid onset of anaesthesia because of its poor uptake into the blood, a high alveolar (and therefore brain) concentration being reached rapidly. On withdrawal from anaesthesia, recovery occurs more quickly with less-soluble agents, which are eliminated from the body more quickly.

The relative potencies of inhalational agents are measured in terms of their minimum alveolar concentration (MAC). This represents the concentration in the alveoli that would be required to anaesthetize half the individuals in an experimental population to a standard surgical stimulus. Lower MAC values thus indicate more potent agents as their effects are achieved with very small concentrations. In contrast, weak agents have a high MAC value. The MAC of halothane, for example, is 0.75%, making it a highly potent anaesthetic agent.

Nitrous oxide

Nitrous oxide has a long history of use in anaesthesia. It was first employed clinically in 1844 by the dentist Horace Wells in the USA. After that, it was used as an anaesthetic agent on its own to induce unconsciousness – so-called 'blue gas', which relied on hypoxia for anaesthesia. More recently and more safely, nitrous oxide has been employed with oxygen as a carrier gas for the volatile agents used to produce anaesthesia. Entonox, a premixed combination of 50% nitrous oxide and 50% oxygen, is used to produce analgesia in obstetrics, by ambulance personnel, in accident and emergency departments and on some hospital wards for dressing changes.

Cylinders of nitrous oxide in the UK are coloured blue. At room temperature, it is a colourless gas, but under pressure it exists as a liquid. Cylinders of nitrous oxide are pressurized to 54kPa × 100 (800 psi) and contain a mixture of liquid on the bottom and gas on top.

Nitrous oxide is poorly soluble in blood, with a blood gas solubility of 0.47 at body temperature. This low solubility means that it is rapidly taken up in the lungs and equilibration between the alveoli and the brain is reached very quickly, making induction rapid. Recovery is also fast because of the excretion from the lungs.

Nitrous oxide is not a potent anaesthetic agent: it has an MAC of 105%, which cannot be obtained under normal clinical conditions. Unconsciousness may be produced by 80–90% nitrous oxide in healthy individuals, but this will not provide surgical anaesthesia. Despite being a weak anaesthetic agent, nitrous oxide is an excellent agent for sedation and can be used in a concentration of up to 70%, that is, with a minimum of 30% oxygen. It produces, in addition to sedation, analgesia, which may alleviate the need for local anaesthesia for some procedures.

The mechanism of action of nitrous oxide is unclear; there is some evidence that the drug may have effects on either opioid and/or GABA receptors. Nitrous oxide is not significantly metabolized and can be used safely on patients with liver or kidney disease. It has little effect on the respiratory system, being non-irritant and causing no increase in secretions or bronchospasm. The cardiovascular effects of nitrous oxide are not significant in the healthy patient, but it does cause direct myocardial depression, which may be important at high doses in people with cardiac failure.

Sevoflurane

Sevoflurane is a relatively new anaesthetic agent in the UK, although it has been used in Japan for some time. It has an MAC of 2.0 and a very low blood gas solubility. These physical characteristics make sevoflurane a potent anesthetic agent, with a rapid uptake and speedy recovery. It is used extensively in day case surgery, for which the rapid recovery is a distinct advantage. Sevoflurane is pleasant to breathe, being non-pungent and non-irritant, and is used for the inhalational induction of anaesthesia in children.

The features that make sevoflurane a useful anaesthetic agent also make it an excellent agent for sedation. Much smaller concentrations are used for the latter indication: 0.1–0.5% compared with up to 5% for anaesthesia. A specially designed vaporizer is required to provide these low concentrations, and the carrier gas is oxygen. The main disadvantage of sevoflurane is that it is partly metabolized, so care is required in people with liver or kidney disease. It is currently not widely used for sedation as vaporizers are costly and more research is needed into its use on patients rather than volunteers. Another agent, desflurane is being introduced into anaesthetic practice; this has the advantages of sevoflurane but is metabolized to a lesser extent.

Local anaesthetic agents: lignocaine

Lignocaine (lidocaine) is one of the most widely used local anaesthetic agents. It is commonly used to provide topical analgesia for endoscopy, in addition to being used for regional anaesthesia in surgery, for postoperative pain relief and as a topical agent to reduce the pain of venepuncture.

Lignocaine is an amide local anaesthetic with a three-part structure: a hydrophilic amino terminal, an intermediate chain and a lipophilic aromatic terminal. This structure gives lignocaine the necessary properties to be an effective local anaesthetic. The hydrophilic portion means that the molecule is water soluble and can be dissolved in a solvent to allow injection, whereas the lipophilic portion allows the molecule to cross the lipid sheath that covers nerve fibres.

Lignocaine's site of action is the nerve membrane. Nerve impulse transmission results from depolarization associated with a change in permeability of the cell membrane to sodium ions, leading to an influx of ions into the nerve cell. This alters the resting potential of the cell, and the impulse is propagated. Lignocaine and other local anaesthetic agents act by preventing the influx of sodium ions and preventing the propagation of the impulse. The blocking of the sodium channels is reversible, and the duration of action varies between different agents.

The onset of action of lignocaine is rapid and the duration of action intermediate compared with other agents. It is a weak vasodilator, and its action is terminated by the blood washing it away from the nerve for metabolism by liver amidases. To prolong the nerve block, lignocaine is often mixed with a vasoconstrictor, adrenaline (epinephrine), which can double the length of action.

Lignocaine is available in a number of different preparations depending upon how it is to be used. It is available for injection in a range of concentrations, as Emla cream and as a 4% spray for laryngotracheal analgesia. The onset of action following topical application is up to 5 minutes, the duration of action being 15–30 minutes.

The adverse effects of lignocaine may result from systemic toxicity, drug interactions or hypersensitivity. Systemic toxicity occurs when a high plasma drug concentration is reached, possibly from exceeding the safe maximum dose or from accidental intravascular administration. Toxic effects include tinnitus and perioral paraesthesia at low levels and, at higher levels, convulsions, direct cardiovascular depression and coma. A suggested safe maximum dose is 4.4mg/kg, but care must be taken to avoid accidental intravascular injection in all patients and to reduce the dose used in patients with cardiac disease.

There is a risk of myocardial depression if lignocaine is used concurrently with beta-blockers and antiarrhythmics. Some drugs (for example, cimetidine) may increase the chance of toxicity as a result of inhibiting the metabolism of lignocaine. Since many individuals presenting for endoscopy are taking these and other drugs, care must be taken if throat spray is to be used. Although there is no direct interaction between sedative agents and local anaesthetics, the patient must be warned before sedation if lignocaine spray is to be used as the effect of numbness in the throat and an apparent inability to swallow can be very distressing.

Further reading

Aitkenhead AR, Smith G (Eds) (1990) Textbook of Anaesthesia, 2nd edn. Edinburgh: Churchill Livingstone.

McCaughey W, Clarke RSJ, Fee JPH, Wallace WFM (eds) (1997) Anaesthetic Physiology and Pharmacology. Edinburgh: Churchill Livingstone.

Whitwam JG, McCloy RF (Eds) (1998) Principles and Practice of Sedatio,. 2nd edn. Oxford: Blackwell Scientific.

Wood M, Wood AJJ (1990) Drugs and Anesthesia, 2nd edn. Baltimore: Williams & Wilkins.

CHAPTER 3

Patient assessment

PAUL MADIGAN

The extending role of the nurse is now a recognized feature of the delivery of healthcare in the UK. The aims of this chapter are to focus on the systematic assessment of patients in preparation for successful endoscopy and to evaluate the special role of the nurse endoscopist in this area. It will address both physiological and psychological aspects of patient evaluation, with a particular emphasis on:

1. taking a medical history;
2. physical examination;
3. contraindications to endoscopy highlighted by patient evaluation;
4. patient education;
5. preparing the patient for the procedure;
6. aftercare following endoscopy.

Within any health setting, it is important for patients to understand why they are attending a clinic and what is involved during a consultation. An introduction will be made, ensuring that the patient understands the concept of nurse endoscopy as many will traditionally expect to see a doctor. Patients who wish to see a doctor should be offered the opportunity to do so, but this may be limited by time constraints and availability. The nurse's communication skills and confident manner can often help to reduce anxiety relating to the procedure and the potential outcomes.

Throughout the chapter, the importance of safe practice and how this might best be facilitated are stressed. This is never more apparent than with the sedated patient, who may be at particular risk. Endoscopy is perceived by some patients as an unpleasant experience, and sedation may be given to alleviate anxiety, aid compliance and produce some degree of amnesia while performing a safe procedure in a conscious patient. The use

33

of sedation may, however, result in both cardiac and respiratory depression, and it should be recognized that there is a low mortality rate in sedated patients undergoing endoscopy. Conversely, inadequate sedation may result in patient distress, lack of compliance or an adverse response to the stress of the procedure.

Patient assessment clearly falls into two areas from the point of view of the nurse endoscopist. When there is space and time, a proper and formal assessment, including a full history and examination, can be made, usually within the outpatient facility or pre-admission clinic. Although this clearly represents an excellent patient care scenario, it is more often than not unrealistic as patients for endoscopy are referred from many clinics and colleagues. The endoscopy practitioner will usually meet the patient for the first time in the endoscopy unit and will have to make a rapid but competent assessment of the patient's fitness for endoscopy using the protocols under which the particular endoscopist works. Nevertheless, a review of the process of patient assessment is useful, if only to highlight areas about which essential information can be obtained.

This fuller assessment will be described first to allow practitioners to assimilate the whole assessment process within their plans. The more limited assessment process possible within the endoscopy unit prior to the procedure is then also outlined, but even this more truncated assessment must take into account all those points that would be raised in a fuller assessment.

Planning for endoscopy

The key to safe endoscopy is good planning. Published data indicate that pre-procedure patient evaluation not only reduces the risk of adverse outcomes, but also improves patient satisfaction (American Society of Anesthesiologists, 1996). Planning is vital as it allows the endoscopist and the endoscopy unit to prepare for the individual needs of the patient, hopefully reducing any potential complications.

The first stage in this process is the referral for endoscopy. This should include not only the indication for the test, but also key details of the patient's medical history. Time constraints and workload may prevent in-depth assessments of the patient's physical and psychological needs being carried out on the day of the procedure, so the clinician can help by supplying such information. Many endoscopy units have established direct referral systems in an attempt to improve efficiency and reduce outpatient waiting times. In such cases, a user-friendly, standardized direct referral form may be utilized. Such forms may employ a tick-box format and highlight relevant information such as the reason for referral, signs and symptoms. Other information should include past medical history, particularly major illnesses affecting the cardiovascular and respiratory systems, and drug history. It is also important to make available the results of any relevant prior investigations.

The next opportunity for patient assessment may well be on the day of the endoscopy itself. Many endoscopy units utilize check lists and nursing documentation, and this may highlight details pertinent to the endoscopist. It is of vital importance that such information is relayed to the nurse performing the test.

Finally, the endoscopist should discuss with the patient the indications for the test, together with a quick résumé of other medical details. This assessment may best take the form of directed questions addressing past medical history, particularly cardiorespiratory disease and coagulation problems. Drugs being prescribed may indicate concurrent medical conditions. The information obtained may highlight relative or absolute contraindications to endoscopy. It cannot be stressed strongly enough that if the information obtained from the patient assessment suggests that the procedure is likely to compromise the patient's well-being, the nurse must be prepared to cancel or delay the endoscopy pending further treatment or investigation.

Complete patient assessment in the outpatient department or preassessment clinic

A more detailed assessment could be made in the outpatient setting, particularly for patients considered to carry a higher risk, including the elderly, those with cardiorespiratory disease, cerebrovascular disease, liver failure, and the obese (British Society of Gastroenterology, 1991). Some units are exploring the role of nurse-led clinics, which may facilitate a more thorough patient evaluation. Meeting the endoscopist before the test to ask questions and receive all relevant information may help to diminish patient anxiety.

The assessment of the patient starts when he or she enters the room. The endoscopist is able to assess the patient's general condition, including level of anxiety, age, size and mental alertness. It is important to observe for obvious signs of illness such as skin pallor, jaundice and breathlessness, and any disabilities, for example poor vision and limited mobility. Language and cultural differences may also need to be considered; an escort with the patient might indicate a limited level of mobility or a reduced level of understanding. Endoscopy may be contraindicated in unco-operative patients and those with a history of mental retardation or dementia (Minocha and Srinivasan, 1998), but the endoscopy may be necessary and play a vital part in the management of the patient. Encouraging a relative to remain with such patients may alleviate anxiety, aid in the consultation and help when explaining the procedure.

History-taking

The aim of history-taking is to elicit an account of patients' clinical problems by obtaining information that is relevant not only to their physical, but also their social and psychological, needs. The history-taking may proceed in a particular sequence, many health professionals obtaining details of patients' social and occupational histories before addressing the presenting complaint. The professional may find it productive to allow patients to give a free account of their history but may need to intervene throughout by giving them prompts that encourage information-giving. This chapter does not cover the correct way of taking a patient history, but it will go through the history-taking process and highlight some of the areas that may be relevant to the endoscopy.

Careful and clear documentation is vital and the following formal headings, adapted from *Hutchison's Clinical Methods* (Swash, 1989), may help and can be recorded in the sequence:

1. Age and demographic details;
2. Presenting complaint;
3. History of the presenting complaint;
4. Past medical history;
5. Drug treatment history;
6. Family history;
7. Social history.

Age and demographic details

Age has an influence not only on disease spectrum, but also on the risk of the endoscopic procedure to the patient. Both gastric and duodenal ulcers are more common in elderly people, who also have a higher risk of serious pathology such as cancer. Conversely, it is well accepted that patients under the age of 40 years are unlikely to have a malignant disease. Co-morbid illness is far more frequent in the elderly population, who also do not tolerate sedation as well as the young. Bell et al. (1987) found that the appropriate dose of midazolam is often overestimated in patients over 70 years of age.

Social background is also relevant as it is a potential indicator of lifestyle, diet and exercise. Lower socioeconomic groups have a recognized higher incidence of cardiovascular and respiratory disease. Patient size may act as an indicator of the quantity of sedation drug required at the endoscopy.

Presenting complaint

During the consultation, it is important to establish details of the presenting complaint and its duration. A considerable proportion of the population will experience mild gastrointestinal symptoms at some time in their life, but the clinician should be alerted by symptoms of recent onset that could indicate serious pathology, such as the patient feeling a lump, vomiting blood (haematemesis) or having difficulty swallowing (dysphagia). Recent weight loss is also a good indicator of severity of disease. Other worrying symptoms include a change in bowel habit, rectal bleeding, jaundice and ascites. These can indicate not only the primary spread of a malignancy, but also secondary spread to the liver.

The majority of patients are unlikely to have a life-threatening condition, and only a small percentage of patients presenting to the clinician will have malignant disease. Common complaints in the gastrointestinal clinic may vary, but many patients will attend with symptoms such as pain, nausea, heartburn, diarrhoea and constipation.

History of presenting complaint

As with any symptom, the clinician should look into the complaint in detail. Exploring the nature, severity and character of the symptoms enables the professional to acquire an understanding of the nature of the disease, which will affect the type of management required. The patient often has difficulty distinguishing between symptoms, for example indigestion and chest pain. If the clinician has a suspicion that the pain could be cardiac in origin, appropriate investigations must be carried out to exclude ischaemic heart disease before proceeding with the endoscopy. The serious complications of ventricular tachycardia, respiratory difficulty and hypotension can occur during an endoscopy in the immediate post-myocardial infarction period, so it is advisable to cancel or postpone the endoscopy.

Associated minor symptoms such as headaches, skin rashes and eye problems may also be relevant and should not be ignored. Women should always be asked about their menstrual cycle as irregular or heavy periods are a cause of anaemia, a frequent indication for requesting an endoscopy. The endoscopy may be inappropriate and the clinician can then proceed with another line of investigation.

If there is a possibility of pregnancy, the clinician must consider whether the endoscopy will put both mother and child at risk, especially during the early stages of pregnancy. Some sedatives, such as midazolam, may be safely used in pregnancy, but there is evidence that this carries some risk and they should be used only when necessary (Minocha and Srinivasan, 1998). Certain sedatives should be avoided in mothers who are breast-feeding as they can be excreted in human milk. It is important to establish whether the woman is taking oral contraception as certain drugs may decrease its efficacy, thereby increasing the risk of pregnancy. If it is necessary to give such drugs, the patient should be advised to use additional barrier methods.

Past medical history

Past medical history can highlight or exclude any major disease that might prevent an investigation being carried out. All important illnesses from infancy, and major diseases such as cardiovascular and pulmonary conditions, diabetes, epilepsy, heart valve replacement and operations, should be documented. Patients at risk are not only those with severe disease, but also those with recent acute trauma such as myocardial infarction and women in early pregnancy.

It is particularly relevant to consider infective endocarditis. Patients at risk of this include those with prosthetic heart valve replacements, a history of endocarditis, congenital cardiac malformations, rheumatic and acquired valve disease, hypertrophic cardiac myopathy and surgically constructed systemic pulmonary shunts (Cotton and Williams, 1996). In such cases, many endoscopists recommend prophylactic antibiotic regimens to prevent endocarditis.

If the patient has undergone an abdominal operation, try to establish the extent of the surgery as it may affect the endoscopic findings and also enable the endoscopist to understand the post-surgical anatomy. Furthermore, previous endoscopies should also be considered. Was the patient sedated; if so, how was he or she affected by this? What were the relevant findings, and how did the overall experience affect the patient?

Drug treatment history

The drug history should include details of all drugs currently being taken, including simple analgesics, oral contraceptives and over-the-counter drugs. Adverse drug reactions and hypersensitivities (especially to penicillin) should be recorded as anaphylaxis may occur if these drugs are administered. If the patient is receiving warfarin, the level of anticoagulation should be noted as prolonged blood clotting will increase the risk of haemorrhage following the procedure, particularly if biopsies are taken.

It is relevant to ask about any history of drug abuse or current use of sedatives and/or hypnotics, which may increase the risk of oversedation, potentially leading to respiratory complications during endoscopy. Establishing the treatment history also enables the clinician to discover what medication has been effective in the past and what might be useful in the future. Drugs may highlight a disease that has not been uncovered in the history but may increase the risk during endoscopy. The use of non-steroidal anti-inflammatory drugs (NSAIDs), for example, may indicate that the patient has arthritis; if this affects the neck, it may increase the risk of subluxation during the endoscopy.

The interviewer should establish whether the onset of symptoms was associated with the use of medication. It is well established, for example, that one of the major causes of peptic ulcer disease is drug treatment with NSAIDs or aspirin; both can now be purchased 'over the counter' and may appear innocuous to the patient.

Family history

Some disease processes have a familial association, so it is relevant to record the state of health, important illnesses and cause of death of the immediate relatives. In the gastrointestinal clinic, the main concerns are malignancies such as gastric and bowel cancer. A family history of a malignancy may raise patient anxiety and have an important impact on the way in which symptoms are manifested. An appreciation of this, and an empathic response, is essential for a satisfactory patient consultation. A family history of heart and lung disease, hypertension or diabetes may also be relevant: these conditions may increase the risk of sedation during the endoscopy.

Social history

The patient's adaptation to work and social background may have repercussions on his or her health. Illnesses, both physical and mental, may relate to an occupational hazard, and the clinician should be aware that chronic illness may result from previous employment, a good example being the lung disease seen in coal miners. Home circumstances and an inability to cope with everyday activities such as cleaning and washing will give the clinician an idea of the extent of any disability and reflect the severity of the disease process. The clinician should ask whether the patient gets out of breath or develops chest pain when attempting these minimal activities as this is an indication of the severity of cardiorespiratory disease.

Food, alcohol, cigarettes and other drugs have important implications in relation to heart and lung disease and psychological instability. Patients who smoke give a fairly accurate account of their tobacco consumption, although alcohol history is often unreliable. Smoking can reflect the degree of lung disease, and alcohol consumption can highlight the possibility of liver damage. The endoscopist should be aware that the amount of drinking and smoking can also influence the dose of sedative required: patients who smoke and have severe lung disease may need only a low dose of sedative, whereas those who have a history of alcohol abuse may require a substantial amount of sedative to induce sleep. The endoscopist can titrate the dose of sedation to the individual needs of the patient, thus enhancing safety during the procedure.

Physical examination

It has been estimated that 90% of gastrointestinal diagnoses are first suggested by the history and the other 10% by a combination of physical findings and investigation results. We will now address the physical examination, which may help to establish a potential diagnosis and also assess the safety of endoscopy for that patient. Briefly, this will include examination of the heart and lungs, evaluation of the airway and abdominal assessment. Good general texts on patient examination include *Clinical Examination* (Epstein et al., 1999) and *A Guide to Physical Examination* (Bates, 1995).

The clinician should observe the patient's demeanour in the early stages of the consultation and then ensure that the patient is positioned comfortably for the physical examination. An initial look at the hands may show indicators of lung and cardiac disease such as clubbing of the fingernails and peripheral cyanosis. The examination can then progress as follows.

Cardiovascular system

The most important signs in the cardiovascular system are pulse and blood pressure. Tachycardia (a pulse rate of more than 100 beats per minute) combined with hypotension (a systolic blood pressure of less than 100 mmHg) indicates shock, which can have many causes. If the patient is shocked, endoscopy is unsafe and should be postponed until the patient has been adequately resuscitated.

The rate, rhythm, character and volume of the pulse should be noted. A rapid heart rate may simply mean that the patient is anxious, but it may indicate a tachyarrhythmia such as atrial fibrillation or suggest thyrotoxicosis. A slow heart rate may be seen in a fit and healthy patient, or it may represent a cardiac arrhythmia such as a heart block or even suggest that the patient is receiving some medication that is slowing the heart rate, for example a beta-blocker.

Blood pressure should be viewed in relation to patient age. A high blood pressure often results from patient anxiety. If the blood pressure remains elevated, the test may need to be postponed.

The clinician should note the height of the jugular venous pressure, seen in the neck. An increase may indicate right-sided heart failure or a rise in circulating blood volume, as with the overadministration of intravenous fluids. Arterial pulsations may be observed in the neck in the anxious patients and those with thyrotoxicosis, high blood pressure or an aneurysm of the aorta. All of these may increase the risk at endoscopy.

Next one should inspect and palpate the precordium, paying special attention to locating the apex beat. This is normally situated in the fourth intercostal space along the mid-clavicular line; it can be displaced in heart failure or ventricular aneurysm. An inability to feel the apex beat may result from obesity or an overinflated chest, as in obstructed airways disease.

Auscultation of (listening to) the heart with a stethoscope should identify the normal heart sounds and any additional heart sounds and murmurs. Valvular heart disease may be discovered, necessitating further investigation before proceeding with the endoscopy. Additional cardiac investigations may include an ECG and echocardiography. The ECG will exclude ischaemic heart disease and the echocardiogram will assess the heart valves and muscle function. A routine ECG is not required in patients who do not have cardiovascular disease, but if at any stage before or during the endoscopy the patient complains of sudden chest pain, an ECG should be performed to exclude ischaemic heart disease and cardiac arrhythmia. If the endoscopist is unable to interpret the ECG competently, he or she should seek the advice of a suitably qualified colleague before continuing with the endoscopy.

Respiratory system

Although endoscopy-related deaths are rare, it is recognized that respiratory depression induced by the effects of sedation is a common contributing factor; examination of the respiratory system is thus a vital part of patient assessment. Even though most patients attending the endoscopy unit will be free from severe lung disease, the administration of the sedative may cause respiratory depression even in those individuals who appear well.

Patients with obstructive airways disease may have a deformed chest and be seen to utilize their accessory muscles of respiration. An increased respiratory rate may indicate respiratory distress or simply anxiety. Central cyanosis may be noted from an inspection of the lips and tongue and indicates significant hypoxaemia.

A gradual deepening and diminishing respiratory effort and rate may be noted in severely ill patients, this respiratory pattern being called Cheyne–Stokes breathing. If such breathing is seen, the patient is probably not fit for endoscopy and should be referred for prompt medical attention.

Chest expansion is only infrequently measured but can highlight asymmetrical lung disease such as a pneumothorax, fibrosis or extensive consolidation. The chest should be palpated, determining the position of the trachea and apex beat: a deviation of these sites may indicate underlying lung disease.

Percussion of the chest should compare the degree of resonance over both lungs as a difference in percussion note can indicate underlying pathology. A hyperresonant note is seen over a pneumothorax, whereas dull percussion notes are caused by pleural effusions, pleural fibrosis and collapse consolidation of lung tissue.

Auscultation should be performed to listen to the breath sounds, which should be compared between the two lungs. Added sounds such as pleural rubs, wheezes, crepitations and crackles may be found, which may suggest pleurisy, asthma, pulmonary oedema and infection respectively.

If any of these signs are identified, the endoscopist should consider their relevance before proceeding with the endoscopy. It may be advisable to postpone the procedure until the patient has been treated or a more experienced practitioner is available. Additional investigations such as a chest X-ray may provide further evidence of the condition of the lungs.

Abdomen

The endoscopist should be able to assess the abdomen for contraindications to endoscopy and be able to recognize signs indicating possible complications after endoscopy, such as perforation of the bowel. A systematic and unhurried examination of all areas of the abdomen will also reassure the patient and help to reduce any anxiety.

Inspection of the abdomen can highlight swelling or distension, which may occur with intestinal obstruction or ascites. Visible peristalsis may be observed in obstruction of the bowel, high-pitched sounds being heard on auscultation. An inspection of the skin of the abdomen will identify surgical scars and distended veins.

Palpation is an important part of the abdominal examination. The clinician should be aware that the patient may have abdominal tenderness so should warn the patient of what is about to happen. It is important to assess muscle tone and to feel for the major abdominal organs as well as any abnormal masses. Pulsations may be found in the epigastrium and can be normal. An expansile swelling in this region may, however, be caused by an aneurysm of the abdominal aorta, and it would be prudent to investigate this before proceeding with the endoscopy.

Percussion will help to outline the position and size of the major organs, the percussion note typically being dull over these sites. Obstructed, distended bowel is occasionally hyperresonant. Free fluid in the abdomen leads to a dull percussion note, which shifts with the patient's position.

On auscultation, the bowel sounds are either present or absent; if present, this could indicate peritonitis. Bowel sounds may, if heard, be normal or increased in bowel obstruction.

The endoscopist should be able to identify the patient with an 'acute' abdomen, who may require emergency surgical intervention. The differential diagnosis of an acute abdomen is extensive, the management varying according to the diagnosis. Signs of an acute abdomen include abdominal tenderness, involuntary guarding (tense abdominal muscles) and rigidity of the abdominal wall muscles. Rebound tenderness is another sign, which indicates peritoneal inflammation. The acute abdomen may also produce shock (see above). Some patients, including the elderly and some people receiving immunosuppressive therapy, may have peritonitis with very few signs.

If the patient gives a history suggestive of colorectal disease, the clinician should perform a digital examination of the rectum.

Investigations

After taking the history and examining the patient, the clinician should review any relevant investigation results. A chest X-ray may highlight chronic lung disease and acute infection but is not routinely necessary before proceeding with endoscopy.

Radiological findings can be important as these may direct the endoscopist towards preparing for a therapeutic endoscopy. Many therapeutic procedures require a more expert and experienced endoscopist and specialized equipment. For example, a barium swallow may highlight an oesophageal stricture, which may require oesophageal dilatation and fluoroscopic screening during the procedure. Findings also enable the endoscopist to plan for a prolonged procedure requiring an increased dose of sedation. Previous blood results may highlight conditions such as anaemia, clotting deficiencies and renal impairment.

Once the clinician is satisfied that the endoscopy is required and no major contraindications have been uncovered by the history, patient examination and ancillary investigations, he or she should ensure that the patient has a full understanding of the procedure. If the clinician feels that the patient will be put at unnecessary risk, the test should not go ahead; some endoscopies, including therapeutic and prolonged procedures, particularly in high-risk patients, carry a greater risk than others.

Assessment immediately prior to endoscopy

It is assumed that a full and proper assessment has been made of the patient in the outpatient or preadmission clinic by a nurse practitioner or medically qualified member of staff to ascertain the patient's fitness for the procedure. A considerable time may, however, have elapsed between this initial assessment and the actual endoscopy appointment, so it is crucial that the situation be critically re-examined immediately prior to the endoscopy.

History-taking

It is usually sufficient to ascertain that the patient still has or is suffering from the complaint that was originally presented at the outpatient clinic. If, however, the history has significantly changed or the patient is no longer suffering from the complaint originally presented, a reassessment of the indications for the endoscopy is probably prudent. There are some circumstances in which this is entirely appropriately carried out by the practitioner at the time, but in other cases it may require discussion with the referring team, and it may even be appropriate to cancel the endoscopy for further discussions and reappointment.

It should be remembered, however, that there are many conditions that are intermittently symptomatic and may still represent serious disease; in such circumstances, and unless there are significant contraindications to the procedure, the planned procedure should be undertaken. This might occur with gastric ulcer-type symptoms in those patients over 50 years of age who have been treated for hyperacidity and whose symptoms have resolved. This treatment may, in some of these patients, have resolved the symptoms of a gastric malignancy, so the procedure should go ahead in this age group. The symptom of rectal bleeding can also be intermittent, and if the history represents a high risk of significant pathology (dark red bleeding, a positive family history, age over 50 years and a previous medical history of polyps or gastrointestinal malignancy) it may again be entirely appropriate to go ahead with the endoscopy even though the patient is currently symptom free. If there is any doubt, the original physician should be consulted.

Drug treatment history

It is important to review patients' current medication as this may change with time and may have been altered by the GP since the original outpatient consultation. The introduction of anticoagulants, NSAIDs, other anti-inflammatory drugs or steroids is important.

Examination

It is not usually necessary to undertake a second complete physical examination, but there should be a cardiovascular assessment in relation to any previous history of a cardiovascular complaint. A routine assessment of pulse and blood pressure should be undertaken prior to the endoscopy. Any alteration in respiratory status, especially in patients with known chronic obstructive airways disease who may have suffered exacerbations waiting for the procedure, should also be noted; a useful hint of this is often obtained by a change in medication for these diseases. Any significant alteration may be important in relation to the risk factors associated with the sedation rather than the endoscopy.

Final risk assessment prior to endoscopy

The American Society of Anesthesiologists (ASA) assessment of risk is easily adapted for use immediately prior to endoscopy, the scheme dividing patients into five categories (Table 3.1). ASA category I encompasses essentially normal patients, whereas those falling into grades II and III will be patients with minor-to-intermediate degrees of medical complaints that are not imminently life-threatening and probably pose no immediate risk in relation to endoscopy, obviously taking more specifically into account those relating to the cardiorespiratory system. Patients who fall into category IV do, however, represent a significant risk of complication, from either the procedure or the sedation, and the less-experienced endoscopist should probably ask for a reassessment by more experienced medical personnel before proceeding with the investigation. Patients in grade V have serious and immediately life-threatening complaints and should probably be assessed by a consultant prior to the endoscopy to see whether the procedure is still required, given the high level of risk that will be associated with it.

Table 3.1 The American Society of Anesthesiologists classification of physical status

Class I	The patient has no organic, physiological, biochemical or psychiatric disturbance. The pathological process for which surgery is to be performed is localized and does not entail a systemic disturbance. Examples: a fit patient with an inguinal hernia, a fibroid uterus in an otherwise healthy woman
Class II	Mild-to-moderate systemic disturbance caused either by the condition to be treated surgically or by other pathophysiological processes. Examples: non- or only slightly limiting organic heart disease, mild diabetes, essential hypertension, anemia. The extremes of age may be included here, even though no discernible systemic disease is present. Extreme obesity and chronic bronchitis may be included in this category
Class III	Severe systemic disturbance or disease from whatever cause, even though it may not be possible to define the degree of disability with finality. Examples: severely limiting organic heart disease, severe diabetes with vascular complications, moderate-to-severe degrees of pulmonary insufficiency, angina pectoris, healed myocardial infarction
Class IV	Severe systemic disorders that are already life-threatening, not always correctable by operation. Examples: patient with organic heart disease showing marked signs of cardiac insufficiency, persistent angina or active myocarditis, advanced degrees of pulmonary, hepatic, renal or endocrine insufficiency
Class V	The moribund patient who has little chance of survival but is submitted to operation in desperation. Examples: burst abdominal aneurysm with profound shock, major cerebral trauma with rapidly increasing intracranial pressure, massive pulmonary embolus. Most of these patients require operation as a resuscitative measure with little if any anesthesia

A record of the assessment process in the endoscopy department is very important. Various structures for documentation have been utilised. The most important factors to be considered are that the record allows the endoscopist/sedationist to quickly and clearly identify potential aspects of risk as highlighted by the assessment.

Patient education, information and consent

Ideally, all these issues below should be discussed before the patient is sedated. Guidelines are included here and are discussed elsewhere in more detail.

Education and information

Clinicians should explain to the patient, in simple terms, any findings from the consultation. They should agree with the patient an action plan of the investigations and treatment required; involving the patient at this stage will hopefully improve compliance. Pre-procedural counselling has been shown to improve patient satisfaction and reduce risks. It is natural that the patient will be anxious, maybe because of the unknown diagnosis or as a result of misguided remarks from friends and relatives on the unpleasantness of endoscopy. The communication skills of the nurse endoscopist can be used to reassure the patient.

The endoscopy should be explained in a friendly, empathic manner. Encouraging the patient to ask questions and allowing time for an explanation will make the patient feel at ease. If the patient has had a previous endoscopy, establish whether he or she was able to tolerate the procedure without sedation. If sedation was given, ask whether the patient remembers the procedure and whether there were any complications, for example a reaction to the sedative. A history of problems does not necessarily mean that sedatives cannot be administered or the endoscopy carried out. The endoscopist may wish to reduce or adjust the sedation required in an attempt to minimize risk (Zuccaro, 2000).

Emphasize the need for the endoscopy and reassure the patient that the procedure is safe and that the patient will be made as comfortable as possible. Giving the patient written information explaining the procedure, perhaps sent out a few days before the test, will support the verbal explanation and allow the patient to give informed consent. This information should explain in simple terms what will happen before and after the test, and include preparation for the endoscopy. The patient should be told when to stop eating and drinking and what medication can and cannot be taken; this may concern many patients, for example diabetics, who have a regular daily routine. A contact telephone number should also be provided. If sedation is to be administered, check that the patient is accompanied as he or she should not drive afterwards. Patients should also understand that they should not operate machinery for 24 hours after endoscopy and sedation.

Informed consent

Informed consent should be obtained before the endoscopic procedure and is normally obtained on the day of the endoscopy. The clinician should tell the patient the reason for the endoscopy, explain the procedure in full and explain the possible complications, which range from the simple and common, such as excessive wind, to the more serious and rare, for example bowel perforation. Alternatives to the procedure should be described and offered, the clinician explaining that these may be less suitable in giving a specific diagnosis.

Consent is detailed elsewhere, as is monitoring the patient during endoscopy.

Post-procedural information

It is common, because of the amnesic effects of the sedation, for the patient not to remember the procedure and retain verbal instructions. When the patient is fully conscious, the endoscopist or nursing staff should explain the endoscopy findings and any recommended treatment regimens that may be required. This explanation may be supported by written information describing the condition and recommended treatment. Written discharge instructions emphasizing the care and precautions required after sedation should be given to patients and those accompanying them. These instructions should contain information on potential complications and how to recognize them, when to resume diet and medication and when to return to normal physical activities such as driving and work.

Patients may be relieved and relaxed at this stage, reporting that the endoscopy was not as unpleasant as they had imagined or been told by their friends. From the clinician's point of view, it is very satisfying that the patient's recovery has been uncomplicated and that the care given has been of a high quality.

References

American Society of Anesthesiologists (1996) Practice guidelines for sedation and analgesia by non-anesthesiologists. A report by the American Society of Anesthesiologists Task Force on Sedation and Analgesia by Non-Anesthesiologists. Anesthesiology 84: 459–71.
Bates B (1995) A Guide to Physical Examination and History Taking, 6th edn. Philadelphia: JB Lippincott.

Bell GD, Spickett GP, Reeve PA, Morden A, Logan RFA (1987) Intravenous midazolam for upper gastrointestinal endoscopy: a study of 800 consecutive cases relating to age and sex of patient. British Journal of Clinical Pharmacology 23: 241–3.

British Society of Gastroenterology (1991) Recommendations for standards of sedation and patient monitoring during gastrointestinal endoscopy. Gut 32: 823–7.

Cotton P, Williams W (1996) Practical Gastrointestinal Endoscopy, 4th edn. Oxford: Blackwell Scientific.

Epstein O, Solomons N, Robins A (1999) Clinical Examination, 2nd edn. London: CV Mosby.

Minocha A, Srinivasan R (1998) Conscious sedation. Digestive Diseases and Sciences 43(8): 1835–44.

Swash M (Ed.) (1989) Hutchison's Clinical Methods, 19th edn. London: Baillière Tindall.

Zuccaro G (2000) Sedation and sedationless endoscopy. Gastrointestinal Endoscopy Clinics of North America 10(1): 1–19.

CHAPTER 4

Clinical techniques

DAVID CRAIG

This chapter describes the practical administration of sedation for endoscopy procedures. Although intravenous midazolam is probably the most generally useful agent, other drugs and routes of administration may occasionally be helpful, so information on these is also provided. Having a variety of techniques at one's disposal makes it easier to manage each patient optimally. In certain circumstances, for example when a patient is allergic to a drug or when venepuncture cannot be tolerated, it may be appropriate to employ an alternative sedation technique. Current sedation techniques employ:

1. intravenous midazolam;
2. intravenous midazolam plus an opioid;
3. intravenous propofol (by infusion);
4. oral or intranasal benzodiazepines;
5. inhalation sedation (nitrous oxide and oxygen).

Sedation using intravenous midazolam

Midazolam (Hypnovel) is a benzodiazepine that is well suited to sedation for endoscopy. It is soluble in water and presented in a 5ml ampoule in a concentration of 2mg/ml, and in a 2ml ampoule in a concentration of 5mg/ml. The more dilute presentation (2mg/ml) is preferred as it is easier to 'titrate', that is, administer in small increments, while observing the patient's response. A titration technique must always be used in order to reduce the risk of overdosage. It is impossible to determine the correct dosage of midazolam by any form of calculation based on the patient's physical characteristics, for example age or body weight.

Clinical effects

Midazolam produces a period of sedation (acute detachment from the individual's surroundings) for 20–30 minutes, this being followed by a state of relaxation for a further hour or so.

Anxiolysis is different from sedation. Anxiolysis (dissolving anxiety) may be described as 'dissociating the patient from the perceived threat'. An ideal sedation drug would be anxiolytic rather than merely sedative as this would leave the patient fully awake and aware of, but completely unconcerned about, what was about to happen. Unfortunately, no such drug exists. It is important to consider the degree of anxiolysis rather than just the depth of sedation when assessing the quality of sedation.

Anterograde amnesia (in relation to sedation) means the reduction in memory recall following administration of the drug. With midazolam, most patients have little or no recall of the operative procedure. Some patients think that they have been anaesthetized rather than sedated; others have difficulty believing that the procedure has already been carried out. This situation must, of course, be fully explained to both the patient and his or her escort before discharge.

Midazolam causes minimal cardiovascular depression. The small reductions in arterial pressure and heart rate seen during midazolam sedation are the result of both direct cardiovascular depression caused by the administration of benzodiazepines, and the reduction in pre-procedural hypertension and tachycardia that is caused by anxiety.

Respiratory depression is seen in all patients undergoing midazolam sedation and is often minimal. There are, however, exceptions, for example patients with impaired respiratory function or those who have been prescribed (or use) CNS-depressant drugs, particularly opioids. Patients may not, of course, admit to recreational drug use/abuse. Overdosage and/or excessively rapid 'bolus' injections often cause profound respiratory depression or even respiratory arrest. The unpredictability of respiratory depression means that a pulse oximeter must always be used whenever intravenous sedation is employed.

Midazolam also has muscle relaxant and anticonvulsant properties, which are generally helpful to the endoscopist. It is important to note that the muscle relaxation often persists for some time and may complicate the patient's management during recovery and the journey home.

The advantages of intravenous midazolam sedation include:

1. rapid onset (3–4 minutes or less);
2. adequate patient co-operation;

3. good amnesia.

The disadvantages are as follows:

1. there is no clinically useful analgesia;
2. respiratory depression occurs;
3. disinhibition effects are occasionally encountered;
4. rarely, there are sexual fantasies;
5. postoperative supervision is needed for a minimum of 8 hours;
6. midazolam is not suitable for sedating children;
7. elderly patients are easily oversedated.

Contraindications

Allergy to any benzodiazepine represents an absolute contraindication to intravenous sedation with midazolam, but benzodiazepine allergy is very rare. A degree of caution is needed in the following situations:

1. pregnancy and breast-feeding;
2. severe psychiatric disease;
3. alcohol or drug abuse;
4. impairment of hepatic function;
5. phobia of needles and injections;
6. poor veins;
7. domestic or professional responsibilities;
8. doubts about the ability to provide a suitable escort.

Hardware

Syringes

The most commonly used size is 5ml, which is ideal for midazolam presented as 10mg/5ml. Some sedationists use the 10mg/2ml concentration and either presentation may be further diluted with sterile water to produce a concentration 10mg/10ml. This has the marginal advantage of making titration easier for sedationists who dislike mental arithmetic as 1ml of solution then contains 1mg of midazolam. The disadvantage of having to mix solutions is that the scope for accidents is increased since water is not the only substance that is presented in clear glass ampoules.

Cannulae and butterfly needles

The *Guidelines for Sedation by Non-anaesthetists* (Royal College of Surgeons, 1993) consider it mandatory for all patients undergoing intravenous sedation to have a flexible plastic cannula placed in a vein in order to ensure continuous and reliable venous access throughout the procedure. The most convenient sizes of cannula for intravenous sedation are between 20 and 22 gauge. The Wallace 'Y-CAN' type has the advantage that blood cannot spill from the proximal end of the cannula as the metal stylet is withdrawn following venepuncture, and the appearance of 'flashback'.

Butterfly needles are no longer recommended for routine use because they are more likely to be displaced through the vein wall should the patient move unexpectedly and they usually become occluded by blood clot 5–10 minutes after administering the sedative drug. Cannulae do not suffer these disadvantages and are no more difficult or painful to insert. Finding a suitable vein for venepuncture may, however, be extremely difficult in some patients, and in these circumstances a butterfly needle may offer the only chance of success, for example when the small and delicate veins on the flexor surface of the wrist are used. Great care must then be taken to ensure that the stainless steel needle does not accidentally 'cut out'.

Other equipment

The following items are also required during midazolam administration:

1. gauze to hold the drug ampoule while it is broken;
2. a straight 21 gauge hypodermic needle for drawing up;
3. a tourniquet (or a suitably trained assistant);
4. a Mediswab for cleaning the skin prior to venepuncture;
5. a stopwatch or watch with a second hand for timing drug increments;
6. non-allergenic tape for securing the cannula;
7. a plaster or small dressing to cover the venepuncture site.

Clinical procedure

In most areas of life, meticulous preparation can greatly increase the likelihood of a successful outcome, and this principle certainly applies when sedation techniques are to be used to make surgical interventions such as endoscopy less threatening. It is particularly important to ensure that the patient is fully prepared for the procedure and that the surgical team is fully prepared for the patient, that is, that all the necessary equipment and drugs are readily available. Nothing is more disconcerting to an anxious patient than having to wait while missing items are located or faulty equipment is replaced. When the patient enters the endoscopy room, everything must be ready so that the sedationist can fully concentrate on putting the patient at his or her ease. Having induced sedation, it is then important that the endoscopist is ready to proceed without delay. A sedation check list helps to achieve this and is also a useful aid for training less-experienced staff.

The clinical environment is also important in putting the patient at ease. Many surgical areas are less than hospitable, and some are frankly alarming. It is important to avoid having 'what to do if a patient collapses' posters and anatomical diagrams displayed within the patient's line of vision and to keep threatening equipment out of site or covered. Someone (possibly another nurse) must offer friendly support when the patient enters the area. Having one person do this is better than relying on the whole team to make the patient welcome: everyone may assume that it is someone else's responsibility.

Before any clinical procedure (including venepuncture) is begun, it is vital to check the patient's name, hospital number and medical history. The blood pressure should have been checked and the patient weighed, and written consent must have been obtained for both the procedure and the sedation. It is also advisable to confirm that the patient has a responsible adult escort who is able and willing to look after the patient for the rest of the day. A patient who is unable to provide a suitable escort must either be admitted for an overnight stay or not be sedated. It is important to be wary of patients who say that they will 'phone a friend' or have arranged a taxi and their next-door neighbour to look after them. These arrangements are seldom satisfactory and may place the patient at risk. If there are any doubts, it is better not to proceed with the use of sedation.

A final check should be made to ensure that the appropriate starvation regimen has been followed, that the patient has emptied his or her bladder and that the patient is suitably attired for the procedure. Note that starvation regimens for sedation may vary between different procedures and endoscopy units.

The following description of administering intravenous midazolam (Hypnovel 10mg/5ml) is appropriate for most fit and healthy adult patients between the ages of 16 and 65. Even within this age group, however, a variation in the response to sedation is common. Patients outside this age range will be discussed later.

The operating table or trolley should be adjusted to the supine position and the patient made comfortable. From the sedationist's point of view, induction is probably most easily carried out with the patient supine, but pre-positioning for endoscopy may be preferred if the patient is large or may present handling difficulties.

Electromechanical monitoring must be established before the patient is sedated in order to establish baseline readings. Pulse oximetry is mandatory. Continuous blood pressure monitoring and an ECG may be advisable for some patients. If supplemental oxygen is indicated, this is the time to apply the nasal oxygen cannulae and turn on the oxygen (2 litres per minute being sufficient).

Venepuncture

A suitable vein must then be found. The most commonly used sites are the metacarpal veins on the dorsum of the hand and the superficial veins of the antecubital fossa, but any large peripheral vein may be used. In patients with poor veins in the upper limbs, it is often possible to use the long saphenous vein in the ankle region or even the small veins on the flexor surface of the wrist. An indwelling cannula should be used for all but exceptional cases.

In order to make the veins more prominent, the venous return from the limb must be occluded either by means of a carefully placed tourniquet or by having an assistant apply a firm (but not too firm) pressure around the circumference of the arm. The limb must be below the level of the heart in order to increase venous 'pooling'. Gentle tapping over the selected vein causes local vasodilatation, which also helps the vein to be seen.

The use of topical anaesthetic agents such as Ametop (amethocaine) or Emla (lignocaine and prilocaine) reduces the discomfort of venepuncture, but these creams must be applied some time before venepuncture in order to achieve good analgesia. Emla reduces peripheral vasodilatation so venepuncture may be slightly more difficult.

Assuming that a topical local anaesthetic cream has not been used, the skin may be cleansed with a suitable antiseptic wipe (practices varying here) and the most readily visible and/or palpable vein selected for venepuncture. The sedationist then inserts the cannula into the vein and checks for the appearance of blood within the chamber of the cannula ('flashback'). Aspiration confirms the correct positioning of the cannula, which is then secured with non-allergenic tape.

Venepuncture is a simple clinical skill that has to be acquired. Anyone can do it, but competence and confidence take time to develop, and practice is the only way to become proficient. Everyone who carries out venepuncture regularly has failures so do not be discouraged. Some patients come self-prepared for multiple attempts having had similar experiences in the past. It goes without saying that the patient must receive adequate support and encouragement during what may be rather an uncomfortable ordeal. A good flow of supportive chat is required, and the practitioner must remember to remove the tourniquet before proceeding to the next stage.

Midazolam administration

The prepared drug (10mg in 5ml drawn up into a 5ml syringe) is attached to the injection port of the cannula and injected slowly according to the regimen below. The patient should be warned of a cold sensation at the needle site and as the drug tracks up the arm. Provided the sedationist is sure that the needle is correctly sited, the patient should be reassured that this sensation will pass within a short period of time. The injection must, however, be stopped immediately if pain is felt radiating down the limb as this indicates arterial injection. A completely or partially extravascular injection is usually accompanied by pain and swelling at the site of the injection. In this case, the venepuncture must be repeated, preferably in another limb.

A suitable administration regimen is 2mg (1ml) injected over 30 seconds, followed by a pause for 90 seconds before giving further increments of 1mg (0.5ml) every 30 seconds until sedation is judged to be adequate. Throughout the induction, the sedationist must talk to the patient and watch for any adverse responses, particularly respiratory depression.

The correct dose has been given when there is slurring of speech and/or a slowed response to commands, and the patient exhibits a relaxed demeanour. Ptosis is an unreliable sign when midazolam is used so this should not be used to judge the adequacy of sedation. Some sedationists check the depth of sedation by asking patients to close their eyes and then try to touch the tip of their nose with an index finger; an inability to demonstrate the appropriate level of coordination is believed to indicate that the patient is adequately sedated.

Patients over the age of 65 years often require much lower doses of midazolam. A suggested administration regimen for these patients is 1mg injected over 30 seconds followed by a wait of at least 4 minutes; additional 0.5mg increments are then given every 2 minutes until sedation is adequate. Patients in this age group often need no more than 2mg in order to provide more than an hour of sedation.

Endoscopy may commence shortly after this state has been attained. Approximately 30–40 minutes of sedation time is usually available, and this should be more than adequate for most endoscopy procedures. It is acceptable to top the sedation up from time to time if the procedure is prolonged, but this is not normally necessary during the first 20 minutes. Additional increments of midazolam only need to be small, 1 or 2mg (less in the elderly) usually being adequate.

At the end of the procedure, the patient should be moved on a trolley to a rest area where he or she should remain under the direct supervision of a suitably trained recovery nurse. Outpatients should be discharged into the care of their escorts, who must be given written and verbal instructions (Table 4.1). Patients must not be discharged until they have recovered to the point at which they can stand and walk without assistance. Although most patients will not be fit for discharge until at least 1 hour after the administration of the last increment of midazolam, there is no fixed time limit and recovery staff should be discouraged from 'watching the clock'. Subject to local rules, tea and toast make a pleasant end to the patient's visit.

The patient should rest quietly at home for the remainder of the day and refrain from drinking alcohol, driving or operating machinery for a minimum of 8 hours. It is important to make the escort aware that the patient should be observed for the first few hours and not simply put to bed out of sight.

Monitoring the sedated patient

In addition to checking any electromechanical devices (for example, pulse oximeter or ECG), the sedationist must be constantly aware of the patient's respiration (rate and depth), the presence of airway obstruction, the depth of sedation and the skin colour. A periodic estimation of heart rate and arterial blood pressure may be advisable for some patients.

Respiratory rate is fairly variable (12–20 breaths per minute in adults) but is nearly always reduced during sedation so must be closely monitored. The depth of breathing is also reduced. Apnoea may occur with an overdosage of (or idiosyncratic response to) midazolam. Such side effects are potentially life-threatening if they are not swiftly recognized and treated. Some degree of respiratory depression is probably present in all sedated patients, but serious problems are most likely to occur immediately following induction (see Chapter 7).

Table 4.1 An example of a patient instruction sheet

For your safety please read and follow these instruction carefully:

- *Before sedation: on the day of treatment*

    - Take your routine medicines at the usual times

    - Do not eat or drink for 4 hours prior to your appointment

    - Bring a responsible adult with you, someone who is able to escort you home and then care for you for the rest of the day

- *After sedation: until the following day*

    - Do not travel alone. Travel home with your escort, by car if possible

Pulse oximetry measures the patient's arterial oxygen saturation and pulse rate via a probe that is attached to the finger or earlobe. The pulse oximeter detects changes in the patient's oxygen supply, the oxygen uptake by the lungs and the delivery of oxygen to the tissues via the circulation. It is thus an excellent monitor of both respiratory and cardiovascular function. Correct functioning can, however, be affected by metallic nail varnish or excessive light falling on the probe. An oxygen saturation below 90% should be investigated and the cause corrected (see Chapter 5).

Bradycardia or tachycardia during sedation should also be investigated. The former may be caused by hypoxia or vagal stimulation, whereas the latter is often the result of painful stimuli. Most pulse monitors have an audible alarm that can be set to provide an audible and visible warning if the heart rate falls or rises beyond clinically acceptable levels. The alarm limits set for bradycardia and tachycardia are normally 50 and 150 beats per minute respectively.

Like respiratory rate, blood pressure is variable. Small variations from so-called normal values are commonplace, and the systolic blood pressure is very often raised in anxious subjects faced with an invasive clinical procedure. Well-controlled hypertension is not an absolute contraindication to sedation; in fact, many patients with high blood pressure are better treated under sedation. For elective investigations, however, patients with a diastolic blood pressure in excess of 110mmHg should be investigated before sedation is given.

Reversal of midazolam sedation

Flumazenil (Anexate) antagonizes the action of midazolam, reversing the sedative (but not amnesic), cardiovascular and respiratory depressant effects. Although flumazenil is usually recommended for use only in emergency situations (for example, benzodiazepine overdose), elective reversal may be helpful for some patients, such as those living some distance from the hospital who have to travel home by public transport. In this case, it is imperative that the usual postoperative instructions for intravenous sedation are given and followed.

Intravenous midazolam plus an opioid

Some patients cannot be adequately sedated using midazolam on its own, so in such circumstances it may be appropriate to administer a small bolus of an opioid drug prior to titrating the midazolam. The opioid selected should ideally have a shorter half-life than midazolam in order to avoid prolonged recovery. Pethidine, fentanyl, alfentanil and nalbuphine have all been used, but it should be noted that all these drugs may cause profound respiratory depression and also nausea or vomiting in approximately 30% of patients. Adequate experience in the use of such 'cocktails' of drugs is essential in order to avoid disasters. If possible, it is preferable to use a single drug.

Intravenous propofol by infusion

Propofol (Diprivan) is a potent, short-acting intravenous anaesthetic agent. In subanaesthetic concentrations, it is a reliable and safe drug for intravenous sedation. In comparison with midazolam, recovery appears to be rapid and 'clear-headed', but amnesia is often less profound. There may be a greater degree of anxiolysis than sedation, so patients often appear to be less 'knocked out' than with midazolam, particularly during the first 10–15 minutes of treatment.

Administered by continuous infusion, propofol is more controllable than midazolam, and the depth of sedation may be varied throughout the procedure. It is particularly useful for short (5–10 minute) cases and when prompt recovery is an advantage. The clinically useful properties of propofol result from a very short distribution half-life (2–4 minutes) and an elimination half-life of 30–60 minutes. Diprivan 1% is presented in 20ml glass ampoules containing 200mg of propofol emulsion (10mg/ml). There are few contraindications, but propofol should be avoided if there is known or suspected allergy and with epilepsy. The drug is not currently licensed for paediatric sedation.

In order to reduce the likelihood of pain on administration, a large peripheral vein should be used and/or 1ml of 1% plain lignocaine added to each 20ml ampoule of propofol. A dose of 30mg (3ml) of propofol is given slowly, followed immediately by an infusion at an (initial) rate of 300mg (30ml) per hour. Sedation usually occurs within 1–2 minutes. The infusion rate may need to be adjusted during the procedure, being for example increased at the start and then reduced towards the end. Particular care is needed with procedures lasting more than 30 minutes in order to avoid too deep a level of sedation. Careful clinical monitoring and pulse oximetry is mandatory, although respiratory depression is often less marked than with midazolam.

Patients are usually fit to leave 20 minutes after the termination of the infusion, but the criteria for discharge and aftercare suggested for midazolam should be observed.

Propofol sedation should be used only by those trained in anaesthesia, and the drug must never be administered by the person carrying out the endoscopy procedure.

Oral and intranasal benzodiazepines

Oral sedation is useful if the patient is afraid of needles and will not accept venepuncture. The sedation produced may be adequate for the endoscopy to be carried out or it may then be possible to cannulate the patient and administer intravenous sedation in the normal way. Oral sedation may be contraindicated in patients undergoing upper gastrointestinal endoscopy.

The most commonly used drugs are temazepam (adult dose 30 mg) and midazolam (adult dose 20mg). Temazepam is best administered as an oral syrup, which is reasonably palatable, but midazolam is very bitter and must be added to a strong-tasting fruit juice. Midazolam may also be administered intranasally. A dose of 10mg of the 5mg/ml concentration is usually sufficient and is surprisingly well tolerated. Intranasal midazolam is more rapidly absorbed than oral midazolam.

The management of patients who have received oral or intranasal midazolam is very similar to that used for intravenous midazolam administration. The depth of sedation is similar (albeit rather less predictable), monitoring with pulse oximetry is mandatory, and the discharge criteria are identical.

Although midazolam does not currently have a product licence for oral and intranasal administration, both of these routes are commonly used in other areas of sedation practice, for example accident and emergency medicine and dentistry.

Inhalational sedation with nitrous oxide/oxygen

The use of nitrous oxide and oxygen in subanaesthetic concentrations was popularized as a method of sedation during the late 1940s. Machines designed to deliver a variable concentration of nitrous oxide in oxygen are readily available.

Nitrous oxide has excellent anxiolytic, sedative and analgesic properties with little or no depression of myocardial function or ventilation. Induction and recovery are rapid, and it has a wide margin of safety (see Chapter 2). Three 'planes of analgesia' have been described by Roberts (1990):

Plane I: moderate sedation and analgesia;
Plane II: dissociation sedation and analgesia;
Plane III: total analgesia.

Planes I and II are termed 'relative analgesia' and are clinically useful, but Plane III is approaching general anaesthesia and is therefore unsafe. The variation between individual patients is such that whereas one person may be adequately sedated with 20% nitrous oxide, another may require in excess of 50%. A titration technique of administration is employed in order to avoid the risk of oversedation.

Because of its relatively poor solubility in blood and body tissues, there is a rapid outflow of nitrous oxide across the alveolar membrane when the incoming gas flow is stopped, which may dilute the percentage of alveolar oxygen available for uptake by up to 50%. This phenomenon is called diffusion hypoxia and is prevented by giving 100% oxygen for at least 2 minutes at the end of the procedure.

Equipment

Modern inhalational sedation machines are similar to traditional Boyle's anaesthetic machines but modified so as to make them safe for use by a sedationist.

Nitrous oxide is supplied in a blue cylinder containing both a gas and a liquid phase, whereas oxygen comes as compressed gas in a black cylinder with a white collar. Portable inhalational sedation machines are designed to operate with two nitrous oxide and two oxygen cylinders, one cylinder of each gas being 'in use' while the other is held in reserve and designated 'full'. Only the 'in use' cylinders should be turned on. A pin index system ensures that the nitrous oxide and oxygen gas cylinders cannot accidentally be interchanged. Nitrous oxide and oxygen pressure gauges give an indication of the contents of each cylinder, but whereas the oxygen gauge falls in a linear manner, the nitrous oxide gauge starts to fall only when nearly all the gas has been used up.

The Quantiflex MDM RA machine 'head' comprises flow meters for nitrous oxide and oxygen, a control valve for regulating the total gas flow and a mixture dial for adjusting the percentage of oxygen and nitrous oxide. Modern inhalational sedation machines are incapable of delivering a gas mixture containing less than 30% oxygen and also contain a failsafe mechanism that shuts off the nitrous oxide if the oxygen ceases to flow.

The mixed gases emerge at the common gas outlet, to which the breathing system is connected. There is a 2 litre reservoir bag that is useful for adjusting the total gas flow to an individual patient's minute volume and also for monitoring respiration during treatment. Reservoir bags are made of rubber and are liable to perish, especially in the area of the bag mount (at the neck of the bag) and down the seams.

Although designs vary, all modern inhalational sedation breathing systems comprise an inspiratory tube, a nasal mask and an expiratory tube. Systems for use with 'active' scavenging differ from those for use with the 'passive' removal of waste gases. Active scavenging is achieved by connecting the expiratory limb of the breathing system to a low-power suction device, whereas passive scavenging often involves simply placing the distal end of the expiratory tube as far away as possible.

Nasal and 'full-face' masks are available in a variety of sizes. The former are most suitable for investigations of the upper gastrointestinal tract. Older-style breathing systems must be cold sterilized, but recent improvements in materials makes some newer models suitable for autoclaving.

Before using the inhalational sedation machine the following should be checked:

1   the cylinders: 'full' and 'in use';
2. the pressure gauges;
3. all the connections;
4. the 'flow' and 'mixture' controls;
5. the oxygen flush control;
6. the reservoir bag;
7. the breathing system and range of masks;
8. the scavenging system.

The safety features and ease of operation of the MDM RA machine (or similar) make it ideal for nitrous oxide sedation. Demand-flow devices such as those used for the administration of Entonox (a mixture of 50% nitrous oxide and 50% oxygen) do not allow the titration of the drug against the patient's response so are not suitable. Equipment designed for general anaesthesia is often unnecessarily complicated.

The advantages of inhalational sedation include:

1. a lack of 'needles';
2. easy alteration of the level of sedation;
3. a minimal impairment of reflexes;
4. rapid induction and recovery;
5. some degree of analgesia.

The disadvantages are that:

1. the sedation also depends on good psychological support;
2. the mask may make oral access difficult;
3. postoperative amnesia is variable;
4. nitrous oxide pollution can occur.

The contraindications include:

1. nasal obstruction, for example a cold, polyps or a deviated septum;
2. cyanosis at rest;
3. poor co-operation;

4. the first trimester (12 weeks) of pregnancy;
5. a fear of masks.

Clinical procedure

After it has been checked that the inhalational sedation machine is working and that extra gas cylinders are available (or that piped gases are flowing), the patient is laid supine in the chair and the procedure explained.

The machine is then adjusted to administer 100% oxygen at a flow rate of 6 litres per minute, and the correctly sized nasal (or face) mask is selected. Remember that patients often prefer to place the mask over their own nose rather than have someone else do it. It is important to maintain a steady flow of conversation and encouragement. The oxygen flow rate (minute volume) may be checked by observing the movement of the reservoir bag. If there is under- or overinflation, the gas flow must be increased or decreased appropriately.

Ten per cent nitrous oxide is then added (90% oxygen) and the patient informed that he or she may feel:

1. lightheaded;
2. changes in visual and/or auditory sensation;
3. tingling of the hands and feet;
4. suffusing warmth;
5. remote from the immediate environment.

This concentration is maintained for one full minute, during which plentiful verbal reassurance is given. The concentration of nitrous oxide is increased by 10% for a further full minute (up to a total of 20%) and then in increments of 5% until the patient appears and feels sufficiently relaxed.

Nitrous oxide concentrations of between 20% and 50% commonly allow for a state of detached sedation and analgesia without any loss of consciousness or danger of an obtunded laryngeal reflex. At these levels, patients are aware of operative procedures and are cooperative without being fearful. If, after a period of relaxation, the patient becomes restless or apprehensive, it is probable that the concentration of nitrous oxide is too high.

After the operating procedure has been carried out, the nitrous oxide is turned off and 100% oxygen is administered for 2 minutes to prevent diffusion hypoxia. The patient may then be asked to sit up and will probably be able to walk (with supervision) to the recovery area. Recovery is usually complete within 30 minutes.

Although inhalational sedation may not be optimal for upper gastrointestinal endoscopy, the technique may be useful for colonoscopy or for venepuncture in severely needle-phobic patients.

Nitrous oxide pollution and scavenging

Long-term exposure to nitrous oxide may result in an increased incidence of liver, renal and neurological disease, and there is evidence of bone marrow toxicity and interference with vitamin B12 synthesis that may lead to signs and symptoms similar to those of pernicious anaemia. For this reason, the Health and Safety Executive (1998) specifies a maximum level of 100ppm of nitrous oxide time-weighted over 8 hours. In order to achieve this level and thus keep nitrous oxide pollution to a minimum, scavenging must be employed.

Other inhalation sedation methods

Various combinations of isoflurane, desflurane, sevoflurane and oxygen have been investigated in recent years, but the lack of a suitable gas delivery system has meant that development is slow. Sevoflurane shows most promise.

Patients with medical problems

Medical problems can clearly be managed only if a full and up-to-date medical history has been taken and is available to the sedationist and endoscopist at the time of appointment. Although there are few absolute contraindications to the use of sedation, the presence of intercurrent disease may modify the sedation technique. In some cases, it may be appropriate to consult the patient's medical practitioner or perhaps ask for advice or assistance from an anaesthetist who has sedation experience. Calling for anaesthetic assistance is, however, best carried out before an emergency develops rather than after (see Chapter 7).

Sedation may be affected by any medical problem but the following are the most common areas of concern:

1. myocardial infarction, angina pectoris and hypertension;
2. asthma/chronic obstructive airways disease;
3. liver disease;
4. pregnancy;
5. psychiatric conditions;

6. tobacco and alcohol consumption;

7. medicines.

A patient who has had a myocardial infarction should ideally not be sedated until at least 6 months after the heart attack. As, however, many endoscopies are undertaken in response to acute or potentially malignant conditions, it may not always be possible to postpone the appointment. In such circumstances, it is sensible to speak to the patient's GP and/or any hospital consultants before proceeding. A patient who has an unstable cardiac condition must be sedated only by an appropriately experienced sedationist or anaesthetist. Supplemental oxygen via nasal cannulae is mandatory in such cases.

Stable angina pectoris often represents rather less of a problem providing the sedative drug is carefully administered and hypoxia avoided. Sedation reduces the anxiety level so the patient may be less at risk of experiencing an attack.

Patients with a history of moderate hypertension may be safely sedated as long as the condition is well controlled, prescribed antihypertensive drugs have been taken as usual and the diastolic pressure is not in excess of 110mmHg on the day of the endoscopy. It should be noted that patients with a low blood pressure are more likely to suffer postural hypotension following sedation.

Mild asthmatics respond well to sedation and, as with some cardiovascular problems, sedation may reduce the likelihood of an acute attack by controlling anxiety. Bronchodilators may be used prior to the appointment, and supplemental oxygen is indicated. Severe asthmatics are at risk so sedation by an anaesthetist is preferable.

Liver disease may decrease the rate of elimination of midazolam from the body, which may affect long-term recovery. Short-term recovery, that is, the recovery which is observed in hospital, may, however, be unaffected and this may produce a false sense of security. It is wise to warn escorts that such patients should 'take it easy' for as long as is needed rather than reassuring them that they will have completely recovered in the usual 8 hour period.

There is no drug used for sedation that is guaranteed to be safe throughout pregnancy. Mothers who are breast-feeding should be warned that some sedative drugs, for example midazolam, appear in breast milk so may produce a degree of sedation in their infant, although this may not always be perceived as a totally negative side effect!

Psychiatric conditions are not a contraindication to the use of sedative drugs but the dosage required may be well outside the normal range, and medicated psychiatric patients are often difficult to sedate well. Apart from the wide variation in the amount of drug required, the sedation 'endpoint' is often ill defined and the period of sedation rather short. The same patient may also sedate differently on different occasions even though the amount of drug administered is very similar. The response to flumazenil is often idiosyncratic, and the drug regimen of such patients must be carefully examined. Flumazenil should not be administered to patients who are receiving long-term benzodiazepine therapy.

Excessive smoking can reduce respiratory efficiency to the extent that hypoxia may be seen during intravenous sedation. Supplemental oxygen may be advisable, and treatment may be disrupted by coughing fits. This highlights the importance of obtaining a baseline saturation level before administering sedation (see Chapter 5).

Moderate drinkers present no problem as long as alcohol is avoided on the day of the investigation. Chronic alcoholics may have compromised their liver function to the point at which they may not be able to metabolize benzodiazepines effectively, and this may prolong their recovery from sedation.

Medication can alert the sedationist to undisclosed disease and raise the possibility of potential drug interactions. Some medicines may interact with or potentiate the action of intravenous sedative drugs and prolong recovery time. Other drugs may share metabolic pathways with benzodiazepines and thus delay recovery. Drugs with potential interactions include antidepressants, benzodiazepines, antihistamines, opioid analgesics, alcohol, H2-receptor antagonists, protease inhibitors and erythromycin. None of these drugs, however, represents an absolute contraindication to the use of sedation.

Discreet questioning regarding the use of recreational drugs may yield useful information and alert the operator to the possibility of compromised veins and a positive HIV and/or Hepatitis B or C status.

References

Health and Safety Executive (1998) Occupational Exposure Limits. London: HMSO.

Roberts GJ (1990) Inhalation sedation (relative analgesia) with oxygen/nitrous oxide gas mixtures. 1. Principles. Dental Update 17: 139–46.

Royal College of Surgeons of England (1993) Guidelines for Sedation by Non-Anaesthetists. London: RCS.

CHAPTER 5

Monitoring the sedated patient

JOHN ELMORE

In this chapter, we will explore the reasons for monitoring the sedated patient and the forms that monitoring might take. The concurrent clinical assessment of the patient and the potential hazards of sedation or endoscopic examination will be outlined. This will include a clinical assessment of the respiratory and cardiovascular systems and the associated signs and symptoms of abnormalities. The aim of this section is to provide practitioners with an understanding of the clinical evaluation of the patient's condition during endoscopy. In addition, it will provide an insight into the implications and management of the risks associated with endoscopic procedures and allow practitioners to practise with greater awareness.

As the science of healthcare moves forward, more devices have become available to aid in the clinical evaluation of patients undergoing various procedures. Some of the more commonly used medical devices for monitoring in the endoscopy suite will be examined in detail, and the practicalities of the machinery used will be explored. In addition, the limitations of such devices in terms of clinical assessment will be examined so that the practitioner will have an impression of the validity of data obtained.

Evidence for monitoring

Patients undergoing endoscopic procedures may be at risk of a number of complications, ranging from cardiovascular instability to respiratory compromise (Kost, 1998). Most of these complications are associated with the use of sedation during the procedure and the interrelated CNS depression (Charlton, 1995). The problems associated with sedative agents are well recognized, as are the risks of respiratory compromise (see Chapter 2). Because of this, the sedated patient needs to be monitored.

Other risks have, however, been identified that are related to the instrumentation used to perform the procedure; complications here include aspiration, perforation, bleeding following biopsy or polypectomy, and the stimulation of vasovagal reflexes (BSG, 1995). These risks must also be taken into consideration if monitoring is to be effective.

In addition, Reed & Reilly (1995) state that complications such as hypoxaemic events, normally associated with sedation, have been observed with patients not receiving sedation during endoscopic procedures. Thus, the practitioner must understand that sedation is not the only reason for hypoxaemia and that monitoring in the absence of sedation is also valuable.

Risks such as these have prompted various professional bodies to draw up guidelines for safe practice when monitoring patients undergoing endoscopic procedures. Organizations such as the British Society of Gastroenterology (BSG; 1991, 1995), the Royal College of Surgeons (1993) and the Society of American Gastrointestinal Endoscopic Surgeons (SAGES, 1996) have published recommendations on monitoring patients undergoing such procedures.

Quine et al. (1995) undertook a study that was set across two regions of England and included 36 hospitals. The study analysed 14 149 gastroscopy procedures and identified that the morbidity rate for patients undergoing diagnostic endoscopy was 1 in 200, the mortality rate being 1 in 2000. These rates are relatively high and have been of concern to many authors who have studied this subject. The researchers further suggested that the use of high-dose benzodiazepines, combined with a lack of adequate monitoring, could have an effect on the mortality and morbidity rates. Although this was a single study, it prompted a reaction from the BSG, which referred to it in the 1995 guidelines. The need for careful monitoring during endoscopy is therefore further endorsed by the BSG, which believes this to be a necessity during the procedure (BSG, 1995).

Medical devices

As mentioned above, medical devices can help in the clinical monitoring of patients undergoing endoscopic procedures, but there is no clear evidence to suggest that the use of medical monitoring devices has a significant effect on outcome for the patient undergoing an endoscopic procedure (BSG, 1991). In the light of more recent evidence on morbidity and mortality rates, outlined by the BSG, a lack of monitoring and operator inexperience may be factors contributing to patient outcome (BSG, 1995). The BSG strongly recommends that the mechanical monitoring of blood oxygen level (pulse oximetry) should be considered standard practice perioperatively during endoscopic procedures. Furthermore, it is suggested that, although electrocardiographic monitoring is not indicated for all patients, it should be used in those patients in whom cardiovascular risks have been identified.

Clinical observation

Mechanical monitoring is no substitute for direct clinical observation and should not be considered as such. Monitoring devices are an aid towards, or an enhancer of, the practitioner's assessment of the patient undergoing an endoscopic procedure. The practitioner must decide, based on clinical judgement and the guidelines set down by professional bodies, which monitoring devices are to be used. The information obtained from mechanical monitoring should be incorporated into the larger framework of that clinical judgement. This should be recognised when determining therapeutic interventions based on the data obtained. In the same way, the practitioner must be aware of the limitations of such devices and of when to place faith in the information provided.

Monitoring the patient undergoing an endoscopic procedure should start with a good understanding of the patient's clinical history, current medications and current pathologies. Practitioners should attempt primarily to identify high-risk patients at this stage, which will allow them to focus their attention on avoiding potential problems during the procedure and prepare them to take appropriate action.

Ongoing respiratory assessment

Respiratory assessment should include an assessment of the airway, a direct assessment of the breathing pattern, and the monitoring of any other indirect signs of respiratory insufficiency.

Airway monitoring

Airway patency can be compromised as a result of a diminishing level of consciousness, oversedation or the instrumentation used to perform the procedure (for example, for the aspiration of gastric contents) (BSG, 1995). It is therefore important for the practitioner continually to monitor the level of consciousness (see Chapter 6) along with the patency of the airway. A deepening sedation level can alert the practitioner to possible compromises in airway patency so that action may be taken to promote patency or reverse the effects of the sedation. Constant, vigilant monitoring of airway patency should therefore be practised, clinical signs of airway compromise noted and action taken.

A recognition of airway compromise involves observation and listening skills along with a knowledge of the signs of airway obstruction (Table 5.1). Any increase in respiratory effort should alert the practitioner and, at the very least, lead to closer monitoring. If it is suspected that there are signs of diminished ventilation of the lungs, auscultation of both sides of the chest (using a stethoscope) will be necessary to ascertain whether there is adequate air entry.

Table 5.1 Clinical signs and symptoms of airway obstruction (Kost, 1998)

Increased respiratory effort
Sternal retraction
Rocking chest motion (out of synchronization with respiratory effort)
Inspiratory stridor (harsh, high-pitched inspiratory sounds)
Hypoxaemia
Absence of breath sounds

Airway patency can initially be promoted by appropriate positioning of the patient on the trolley (placing him or her semi-prone with the neck slightly extended), also ensuring that potential hazards to airway obstruction (for example, dentures) are removed. Further means can be utilised, such as lifting the chin upwards (the chin lift) or moving the jaw forwards (the jaw thrust) if difficulties are encountered; in certain circumstances, it may be necessary to pass an oral or nasal airway to maintain a patent airway.

Regurgitation of the gastric contents is a known complication during endoscopy that can compromise the airway. In this instance, the patient is at risk of developing further complications because of damage to the lung tissue. The BSG (1991,1995) recommends that equipment such as tilting beds, supplemental oxygen and suctioning equipment should be available in the event of such an emergency. This will maximize the range of treatments available to patients who regurgitate gastric contents and minimize the risk of aspiration into the lungs. It may ultimately become necessary in such situations to pass a cuffed endotracheal tube to maintain a safe airway and decrease the risk of further gastric aspiration.

Respiratory pattern

Concurrently with airway monitoring, the practitioner should be observing for other signs of effective respiratory function. Breathing should be assessed for rate and regularity prior to, during and after the procedure. A reduction in respiratory rate (bradypnoea) and depth may be induced by sedatives and may be a prelude to respiratory insufficiency. Taking a baseline respiratory rate prior to the procedure will allow the practitioner to make value judgements on any subsequent changes.

A high respiratory rate with an increased depth of breathing (hyperpnoea) may be the result of hypoxaemia and necessitate the administration of supplemental oxygen. Depth of breathing is an important part of respiratory assessment, so practitioners should ensure that they have a clear view of the patient's chest movements during the endoscopic procedure. Depth of breathing, whether the breathing pattern is comfortable or strained and whether the abdominal or accessory muscles are being used are all part of the clinical assessment.

An alteration in breathing pattern may indicate the onset of respiratory insufficiency, so an adequate knowledge of respiratory patterns and their possible implications should underpin the practitioner's understanding. Table 5.2 outlines a list of terms associated with various respiratory patterns and a description of those patterns. A baseline assessment should be made, subsequent assessments being undertaken to determine any change in pattern.

Patients who present with underlying respiratory disease may already show signs of altered respiratory pattern, and this must be part of the initial assessment. Disorders such as obstructive pulmonary diseases (obstructive breathing), restrictive pulmonary diseases (tachypnoea), neurological

Table 5.2 Respiratory patterns (Owen, 1992)

Respiratory pattern	Description
Eupnoea	Normal respiration. 10–16 breaths per minute (young adult); 18 breaths per minute (older adult); rhythm is smooth and even with expiration longer than inspiration
Tachypnoea	Rapid superficial breathing; regular or irregular breathing
Bradypnoea	Slow respiratory rate; deeper than usual depth; regular rhythm
Apnoea	Cessation of breathing
Hyperpnoea	Increased depth of respiration with normal to increased rate and regular rhythm
Ataxic breathing (Biot's respirations)	Periods of apnoea, alternating irregularity with a series of shallow breaths of equal depth
Kussmaul respirations	Deep regular sighing respirations with an increase in respiratory rate
Apneusis	Long, gasping inspiratory phase followed by a short, inadequate expiratory phase
Obstructive breathing	Long, ineffective expiratory phase with shallow, increased respirations

problems (ataxic breathing) and altered respiratory patterns caused by injury (apneusis) can have associated changes in respiratory pattern.

A word of warning should be introduced here: when assessing breathing pattern, not all changes in respiratory pattern are caused by respiratory disorders. Hyperpnoea, for example, can be caused by anxiety or exertion, and bradypnoea can be simply a 'sleep' breathing pattern.

Other elements of respiratory monitoring

Prolonged respiratory insufficiency can lead to severe hypoxaemia, signs such as sweating and cyanosis, along with changes in breathing pattern, being seen. It is to be hoped that the patient will not reach this stage as monitoring devices such as pulse oximetry (discussed in more detail below) will pick up the reduction in blood oxygenation before this eventuality. A knowledge of these end-stage clinical observations should, however, be added to the practitioner's armamentarium, as no piece of equipment is totally reliable.

Cardiovascular assessment

Pulse

An initial assessment of the patient's pulse can offer valuable information (Table 5.3). The rate, strength and character of the pulse can be assessed over the radial artery, changes in these parameters then being further assessed during the procedure. This will also be useful when trouble-shooting, when the functioning of the machinery is in doubt (see oscillometric blood pressure and pulse oximetry monitoring below) and to confirm other clinical signs of deterioration.

Table 5.3 Parameters to assess when monitoring the pulse

Rate
Rhythm
Volume

An initial assessment of rate should be undertaken when the patient is relaxed (not immediately on arrival) and when there is the minimum risk of an increased rate being caused by anxiety or exertion. This baseline value will be useful if tachyarrhythmias (abnormally high pulse rates) or bradyarrhythmias (abnormally low pulse rates) occur during the procedure. The patient may have a low pulse rate that is normal, as in the case of a young, fit, athletic man or woman. A low rate may also result from certain medications such as beta-blockers; this may be picked up from the past medical history. A high pulse rate may be seen simply because people are anxious and/or extremely unfit.

A baseline assessment of rhythm will also be useful as this may indicate an underlying cardiac condition. An irregular pulse rate or missed pulse beats prior to the procedure may identify patients who are currently suffering from arrhythmias. These irregularities may be signs of underlying disease, demanding more careful monitoring. It should also be recognized that certain irregular pulse rates are normal: sinus arrhythmia (a slowing down and speeding up of the pulse during inspiration and expiration respectively) is normal in young healthy adults, and extrasystoles (extra beats) are common without any underlying disease (see below).

Assessing pulse volume along with rate and regularity throughout the procedure can help to determine the quality of the beats reaching the peripheries. Atrial fibrillation is often characterized as a weak (thready), irregular pulse, and this can be induced in patients who are hypoxaemic.

Blood pressure

The estimation of blood pressure can provide valuable information to the practitioner. It can be used to differentiate between normal and abnormal presenting conditions, and also to determine changes in a patient's condition during the procedure. The gauge of what is normal or abnormal blood pressure is difficult to define, and exact definitions are controversial. Swash (1995) quotes normal systolic blood pressure as being 100–140mmHg and normal diastolic blood pressure as 60–90mmHg in healthy adults. He emphasizes that age makes a difference when ascertaining normal blood pressure values and should be taken into consideration: children have normal blood pressures at the lower ends of these ranges, whereas normal values for the elderly lie at the top of, or above, the upper limits of the ranges. The practitioner must use clinical judgement and a knowledge of the patient's past medical history to decide whether the blood pressure recorded can be viewed as normal.

When using changes in blood pressure to ascertain alterations in a patient's condition, it is important to consider the blood pressure in context. When continually monitoring blood pressure, the most valuable information comes from the changes from baseline and from the other elements of the clinical evidence. Observing variations in the patient's condition, and correlating these with blood pressure and changes in pulse rate, oxygen saturation and respiratory pattern, can help the practitioner to complete the clinical picture.

Hypotension

Hypotension has been identified as a risk factor when administering sedative agents (see Chapter 2) as it can also be a direct result of hypoxaemia (Table 5.4). Hypotension is defined as a drop in arterial blood pressure of 20–30% or a systolic of <90mmHg; it may be caused by a variety of factors (Kost, 1998), including:

1. hypovolaemia;
2. myocardial ischaemia;
3. pharmacological agents (such as sedatives);
4. acidosis (more a result than cause);
5. parasympathetic stimulation (pain, vagal response).

In the endoscopy suite, some of these factors may arise directly from the intervention or procedure, such as from excessive bleeding caused by perforation, polypectomy or biopsy, which places the patient at risk of hypovolaemia. Instrumentation and the stimulation of vasovagal reflexes may also cause hypotensive episodes. As sedation and instrumentation can both induce hypoxaemia, acidosis may result and further exacerbate the hypotension. Risks may also occur secondary to other underlying effects of the procedure: myocardial ischaemia may, for example, be a result of

Table 5.4 Physiological effects on the cardiovascular system of acute oxygen lack in healthy adults (Moyle et al., 1994)

Effect	Outcome
Coronary vasodilation Systemic vasodilation Decreased after-load Increased cardiac output Increased stroke volume Tachycardia Systemic hypotension	Can ultimately lead to cardiovascular collapse
Inverted T waves Slowing of conduction Lengthening of P-R interval ST elevation	Changes seen in electrocardiogram
Loss of tone Leakage of fluid	Changes seen in capillaries
Pulmonary vasoconstriction Redistribution of blood to coronary, cerebral, and renal arteries	Other changes

hypoxaemia. The additional effects of hypotension can increase myocardial strain and exacerbate the ischaemia.

Since the patient undergoing an endoscopic procedure is ultimately at risk of all of these occurrences, assessment for hypotension should provide a good indication of the patient's condition during the procedure. In addition, measuring the oxygen saturation will ensure that the practitioner can reduce the risk of undetected hypoxaemia. Peripheral vasoconstriction may be the result of hypovolaemia and affect the probe's ability to obtain a reading (see pulse oximetry below for alternative sites). In this case, close blood pressure and pulse rate monitoring are essential if there is any suspicion that the patient is at risk of excessive blood loss.

Severe hypotension will necessitate medical intervention and should be treated according to its cause, some of the definitive treatments for hypotension (Kost, 1998) being listed in Table 5.5. It is, however, important to emphasize that the practitioner's paramount aim is to prevent hypotension.

Table 5.5 Treatment for hypotension (Kost, 1998)

Administration of oxygen
Administration of fluid challenge
Correction of acidosis
Relief of myocardial ischaemia
Titration of sympathomimetic medications
Titration of inotropic medications

Hypertension

Hypertension may be a direct result of anxiety or exertion, in which case it will be detected during the initial assessment of the blood pressure before the procedure has taken place. Hypertension may also be caused by factors such as anxiety or pain during the procedure, for which analgesia or further sedation may need to be administered.

Hypertension must be taken in context as there is no absolute value at which high blood pressure can be diagnosed as an emergency situation (Shoemaker et al., 2000). It is the relative change in blood pressure values and the possible causes that must be considered, any intervention being considered within this context. It must be remembered that an abnormally elevated blood pressure predisposes the patient to increased bleeding, leads to cardiac arrhythmias and increases myocardial oxygen consumption (Kost, 1998).

As with other methods of monitoring, pre-procedural blood pressure measurements, along with a good clinical history, will help to place the readings in context. Patients with a history of hypertension and those receiving antihypertensive therapies should be monitored more closely. These patients' usual blood pressures will be high, and a reduction to 'normal' levels will in effect lead to hypotension.

A significant increase in blood pressure in those who are normotensive may put a strain on the heart and increase the risk of haemorrhage during the procedure. As with hypotension, it is important first to identify the cause and to treat it accordingly. Table 5.6 lists a set of possible therapeutic approaches to treat hypertension of various causes (Kost, 1998).

Table 5.6 Causes and treatment of hypertension (Kost, 1998)

Fluid overload requires diuresis
Noxious stimuli require analgesia or discontinuation of stimuli
Sympathetic nervous stimulation may require alpha and beta blockade
Myocardial ischaemia may require nitrates and analgesia

Pulse oximetry

Pulse oximetry monitoring is generally an effective and accurate method of determining oxygen saturation in patients undergoing endoscopic procedures. It is recommended by SAGES (1996) as one of the routine methods of monitoring patients during such procedures. It is also recommended for the routine monitoring of all endoscopy patients by the BSG (1991, 1995) as clinical observation is unreliable for detecting early signs of hypoxia or respiratory depression.

How pulse oximetry works

The light absorption spectrum of the haemoglobin molecule changes depending on its level of oxygenation. Oxygenated haemoglobin is redder than deoxygenated haemoglobin and, using this distinction, the level of oxygen saturation in the blood can be estimated. The practicality of applying this is not, however, as simple as it first appears as the tissue structures also absorb light. Thus, any estimate of the relative 'redness' of the blood within the capillaries could be subject to error caused by other sources of pigmentation.

Early instruments heated the area to be measured in an attempt to 'arterialize' the tissue (so more accurate readings could be taken) and measured many wavelengths of light to correlate the information obtained. This method was neither effective nor practical for use in the clinical environment, although some short-term 'perioperative' probes in current use apply the warming principle for greater accuracy. Modern pulse oximetry machines determine oxygenation from the difference in light absorption between each pulse wave on the measured area. By measuring the different light levels, the absorption caused by the tissues can largely be eliminated. This allows for a reduction in error, providing a more accurate reading of the state of oxygenation of the haemoglobin molecule.

The measurements are obtained from two 'light-emitting' diodes, red and infrared, sending pulses of light to a detector in rapid sequence (up to 600 measurements per second). This information is sent to a microprocessor where each measurement is accepted or rejected and weighted using an algorithm (unique to each manufacturer). Once the measurements have been processed, the readings are averaged and displayed to the user. To further ensure accuracy, the information displayed is an average reading based on the set of measurements obtained over the previous 3–6 seconds. In most machines, the strength of the pulse (plethysmography) will also be displayed, either as a linear representation or more commonly as a continuous graphical representation of pulse pressure (Figure 5.1). This information will help the practitioner to gauge the strength of signal being received by the pulse oximeter.

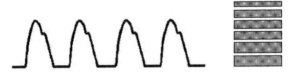

Figure 5.1 Graphical representation of pulse pressure.

What pulse oximetry reads

The saturation of arterial haemoglobin (SaO_2) can be directly measured by obtaining a sample of arterial blood and analysing it in a blood gas analyser (a co-oximeter). Arterial blood is normally between 97% and 99% saturated, but this value can vary depending on a number of factors including age, clinical history and current treatment (such as oxygen therapy). With certain pathologies, such as chronic obstructive pulmonary disease and asthma, the saturation can drop to as low as 85–95%. This emphasizes the need for baseline readings of oxygenation to be taken before performing endoscopic procedures.

Pulse oximetry estimates this parameter without the need for an invasive procedure and normally gives an equivalent value (SpO_2). The accuracy of SaO_2 readings is generally high, the error being reported to lie within 2% with an SaO_2 of more than 70% (Singer & Webb, 1998).

Patients' oxygen saturation can fall during clinical procedures such as endoscopic examination. Hypoxaemia is poorly detected during normal clinical assessment and may become severe before obvious signs manifest themselves: the saturation level can fall to as low as 80% before there are visible signs of cyanosis (Hanning & Alexander-Williams, 1995). The early detection of changes in SaO_2 can therefore be of great clinical value to the practitioner.

Arterial blood gas analysis can be used to calculate the traditional parameter for assessing the effectiveness of oxygenation of the blood, the partial pressure of oxygen in the serum (PaO_2). This gives a good indication of how effectively oxygen is reaching the microvasculature. The relationship between PaO_2 and SaO_2 can also be estimated, thus providing the practitioner with a good insight into patient oxygenation.

The oxygen dissociation curve (see Chapter 2) provides this correlation between the partial pressure of oxygen in the arterial plasma and the saturation of oxygen in the haemoglobin. It is useful to understand this relationship so that the practitioner can be aware of the implication of lower saturation levels. The most notable part of the oxygen dissociation curve is the steep downward slope as the SaO_2 drops below 90%. At this saturation level, smaller reductions in oxygen saturation result in a significant fall in oxygen tension (PaO_2).

Limitations of pulse oximetry

It is important to understand the method used to obtain this measurement in order to gain an insight into why erroneous readings can occur in certain situations. As pulse oximetry depends on the emission and detection of two light sources and the calculation of the differential values of pulsation, there are several reasons why the readings can become inaccurate.

The most common errors occur when there is poor perfusion of or intense vasoconstriction to the area of measurement. This can lead to inaccurate readings ('fail soft') or no readings at all ('fail hard'). More modern machines tend to produce no measurements in this situation ('fail hard') and indicate that an inadequate pulse is being obtained (Singer and Webb, 1998).

Patient movement and/or vibration can interfere with the probe's ability to detect a pulse, and this can result in failure to read the SpO_2 accurately. Intense or excessive ambient light can also inhibit the probe's ability to take accurate readings.

As only two wavelengths of light are used, the instrument is unable to differentiate between oxyhaemoglobin and altered (non-oxygen-carrying) haemoglobin molecules such as carboxyhaemoglobin and methaemoglobin (which have similar light emissions). If these molecules occur in significant quantities in the bloodstream, a false impression of the patient's blood oxygen saturation will be obtained.

Venous pulsation can alter the values recorded, and since a small amount of venous pulsation is normal, there may be a 1–2% discrepancy between finger and ear probes. In disorders such as tricuspid valve incompetence and venous congestion, in which venous pulsation is greater, larger errors may occur.

In addition, certain sources of artificial pigmentation can alter the readings obtained from pulse oximetry. Vital dyes such as methylene blue and indocyanine green can affect values of SpO_2, and even nail varnish has been implicated.

Above all, pulse oximetry is a very poor monitor of respiration especially if the patient is receiving supplementary O_2. A fit patient receiving 40% O_2 can take 3–4 breaths/minute and still record an $SaO_2 > 96\%$ (although their CO_2 will be high). It is only an adjunct to measurements of respiratory rate.

Types of probe and probe placement

Probes come in various designs and are effective for different purposes. Finger probes are the most commonly used. They can be housed in a durable plastic coating, which is easily cleaned, or in a soft coating to improve comfort for longer-term usage. Disposable probes are also available if single usage is necessary, but this has cost implications. Finger probes can, depending on their design, be used on the toes; in some situations, this may in fact be the preferred site. Most manufacturers design their finger probes to exert the minimum pressure on the area being monitored, but when monitoring is prolonged regular changes of site are advisable.

Finger and toe placement can be problematic for several reasons. First, these areas are normally very mobile, which increases the risk of movement artefacts when monitoring SpO_2. Second, the blood supply is likely to become compromised in the peripheral areas before anywhere else if there is vasoconstriction or pre-existing peripheral disease. Most probes should be placed on the finger such that the lead runs along the back of the hand; this stops it becoming entangled with the thumb. In addition, while the hand is resting on a flat surface, the lead can be traced up the arm so that no unnecessary torque (resulting from the effect of gravity) can be applied. There are, however, some probes that are designed to run along the palm of the hand, which highlights the need to read the manufacturer's instructions before probe placement. In the more mobile patient, finger probes that have an adhesive coating can be used to ensure a more secure contact with the area being monitored – these are disposable and, as previously mentioned, have cost implications. Other systems that are single use and have a wrap-round fastener (sensor bandage) are available and are useful for patients who are mobile.

Ear probes are generally recommended for long-term use, but they can be used in the short term if there are problems of peripheral perfusion. Ear probes can be placed on the earlobe or around the pinna. They are designed like a clip and are smaller than finger probes, which makes them less obtrusive and more easily sited in the sedated patient. Self-adhesive, disposable ear probes are also available, which can offer more security to placement.

Other areas of the body can be used if it is difficult to get readings from these sites. The nasal septum, the forehead or even folds of skin can be used to monitor SpO_2. These employ specialist probes, and advice on the advantages of such devices should be sought from the relevant manufacturers.

The site chosen for the readings and the type of probe used can alter the strength of signal and therefore the accuracy of SpO_2 measurements. It is useful to have a small selection of devices available in order to be able to meet individualised needs. One type of probe (usually a finger probe) can, generally speaking, be used for most patients, depending on the choice taken to meet differing clinical areas.

Trouble-shooting

The most common problem with pulse oximetry is poor perfusion to the area being measured, so an initial assessment of the extremities may allow the practitioner to decide which probe to use and where placement is most likely to be effective. This should include feeling for warmth and observing the colour of the area to assess perfusion. It is not always possible to find an ideal site easily, and in such cases trial and error is the most appropriate action to take. If, for example, a finger probe is proving to be unsuccessful, trying alternative fingers or thumbs may resolve the problem. By observing the plethysmograph in different areas, the practitioner can gauge the most appropriate site. Ear probes are often a good alternative if perfusion is poor peripherally.

A patient's clinical history can alert the practitioner to possible perfusion-related problems. Conditions such as heart failure or peripheral vascular diseases may necessitate the use of probes that do not use extremities such as fingers and toes. If a history of heart valve disease is suspected, caution should be taken when interpreting the measurement of SpO_2 as venous pulsation might alter the measurement.

If continuous blood pressure measurements are being taken, the area distal to the cuff will experience intermittent drops in pulse pressure, which will have an alternating influence on the perfusion of that area. The recommendation is therefore not to use the same limb to monitor blood pressure (if performed frequently) and SpO_2 as measurements may be inaccurate or absent.

Movement artefacts are also a common reason why probes fail to read correctly. Some probes will make an allowance for this by increasing the length of time over which the measurements are averaged, but if there continues to be an excessive movement of the area, an alternative site should be considered. Securing the lead to the patient with tape may be an option to reduce the drag placed on the probe by movement. Shivering and tremors will also have an adverse effect on the probe's ability to pick up an adequate signal. This may be resolved by repositioning the probe or, more directly, by addressing the cause of the tremor (for example, anxiety or cold). Similarly, vibration problems can be minimized by identifying the source of the problem and dealing with it or resiting the probe.

Dyshaemoglobins such as carboxyhaemoglobin, often raised in smokers and urban-dwellers or after the direct inhalation of carbon monoxide (suicide attempts and smoke inhalation injuries), can be identified from the clinical history. The only absolute way of differentiating between oxyhaemoglobin and other types of haemoglobin is co-oximetry as this technique measures more of the light spectrum and is a more direct measuring system.

Strong light sources such as surgical lamps may cause errors, and this must be considered in the clinical environment. Simply removing or redirecting the source or, if this is not possible, shielding the probe will solve the problem.

Equipment failure can constitute some of the problems encountered, perhaps requiring a replacement of all or parts of the machinery. The operator should be aware of certain common problems with 'wear and tear', for example damage to cables, especially around the joint between the cable and the probe. Such problems can be pre-empted if care is taken with the equipment. Unnecessary bending of the cables, standing on the cables (increasing the torque on fragile areas) or allowing the cables to be pinched in cot-sides decreases the lifespan of the probes.

Continuous non-invasive blood pressure monitoring

Blood pressure was traditionally monitored using a sphygmomanometer to gauge pressure and a stethoscope to hear the Korotkoff sounds, thus identifying the systolic and diastolic blood pressure. This method of blood pressure measurement is still of value in the clinical setting, but machinery has been developed that can automate this process and thus save the practitioner time by reducing his or her workload. The practitioner must decide which method of blood pressure monitoring suits the particular clinical environment. This may depend on factors such as frequency of monitoring, staff-to-patient ratio, budget and training. As a minimum, however, blood pressure should be measured as a baseline figure prior to endoscopic procedures. There are many machines available on the market that measure blood pressure automatically, most of which give readings that include systolic, diastolic and mean arterial pressure and pulse rate.

Determination of blood pressure by automated blood pressure devices

Automated blood pressure devices initially measured only the mean arterial pressure and lacked sensitivity. In the 1970s, devices were developed that used crystal microphones placed directly over the brachial artery to identify systolic and diastolic pressure as the cuff deflated. Since then, machines have been developed that do not require the precise placement of 'listening' devices. Those in most common use today measure blood pressure in the clinical setting using the oscillometric method.

This involves the machine inflating the cuff to a preset level and decreasing the pressure in steps over a set period of time (Figure 5.2). The machine uses a sensitive transducer to detect the oscillations in pressure as the pulse returns to the limb involved. It is the change in amplitude of these oscillations that allows the machine to determine systolic, diastolic and mean arterial blood pressure. The machine will inflate the cuff to a preset level (170–180mmHg) and will step the pressure down according to predetermined parameters. As the pressure falls, the microprocessor will measure the pulsation at each step, looking for two similar amplitudes. If it detects these, it will move to the next step; if, after a set period of time, it has not detected a pulse, it will deflate. This means that the period of time over which the cuff is inflated depends on the rate and regularity of the patient's pulse.

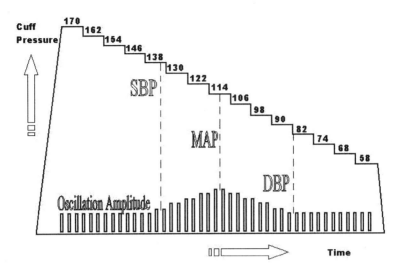

Figure 5.2 Oscillometric blood pressure tracing SBP, MAP, DBP.

As the first Korotkoff sound (representing the systolic blood pressure) is heard, the oscillations increase and the machine can determine the pressure. The oscillations then continue to increase in amplitude, to a maximum, which will denote mean arterial pressure. Finally, the amplitude of the oscillations falls, this denoting diastolic blood pressure.

Correct procedure with non-invasive blood pressure monitoring

As with other non-invasive methods of determining blood pressure, various factors have to be taken into account if the blood pressure is to be accurately determined. Some are similar to those seen when using a sphygmomanometer and stethoscope, but others are unique to using machinery that employs the oscillometric method.

Cuff size (bladder size) is an important factor in the accurate measurement of blood pressure. The cuff circumference should be changed to meet patient size as using the wrong size will give erroneous results: too large a cuff will tend to underestimate blood pressure measurement, and too small a cuff will overestimate it. It is recommended that the cuff bladder should equal the entire circumference of the limb being measured (Stephenson, 1998), but individual manufacturers list recommended cuff and bladder sizes for their equipment, and these specifications should be consulted.

In the case of upper arm cuffs, the cuff should be placed at the midpoint between the axilla and elbow joint, avoiding both of these areas. The cuff should be placed snugly around the circumference of the arm. If the cuff is placed too tightly, there is a risk of inaccuracy of measurement and also associated problems of venous congestion. If it is too loosely placed, readings may be inaccurate or the cuff may become misplaced. Placing the cuff such that you can comfortably slip your finger between cuff and skin represents an ideal tension. When positioning the cuff, all the air must be expelled from the bladder as this can affect the readings and interfere with the machine's internal calibration.

Arm position can, as with the sphygmomanometer, influence the readings obtained using the oscillometric method. The patient's arm should lie roughly at the level of the heart as elevating it will, because of hydrostatic pressure, lead to a fall in the blood pressure measured. The arm should also be left in a neutral resting position and hyperextension of the arm avoided as this can falsely elevate the result. The arm should be supported and the patient encouraged to remain motionless while the readings are being taken. Motion artefacts can interfere with the machine's ability to determine the oscillations properly and necessitate reinflation of the cuff, causing unnecessary discomfort. Some, but not all, manufacturers recommend that clothing be removed in the area of measurement, for example by rolling the sleeve up, as this will alter the readings. It is best to read the manufacturer's instructions before deciding on which policy to adopt.

Prior to placement, the practitioner should assess circulation distally to the cuff as this may become compromised while the measurements are being taken. If frequent measurements are needed, the circulation should be assessed on an ongoing basis and the cuff repositioned if any signs of peripheral insufficiency are observed. As many automated devices can be set at frequent intervals, this is an important aspect of nursing care, and limbs should be kept exposed so that observation is easier.

Most machines will initially inflate the cuff to a preset pressure, but manufacturers are now introducing 'smart' technology whereby, on subsequent measurements, the cuff is inflated just above the previously recorded systolic blood pressure measurement. This is to improve patient comfort as frequent cuff inflations of up to 180mmHg can become unbearable to some patients. Some manufacturers allow the initial cuff inflation pressure to be set by the user; if the practitioner knows the patient's approximate blood pressure, this is a useful way of improving patient comfort.

The cuff should not be placed on a limb bearing an intravenous cannula that is being used for administration of a continuous infusion as it will periodically inhibit venous return.

Hose connectors should be tightened securely but not overtightened. Loose connections will cause a leakage of air and failure to inflate the cuff, whereas overtightening will cause damage.

In the interests of safety, the machine should be placed on a flat surface, attached to a wall or secured correctly to a trolley.

Extras in equipment design

Modern automated blood pressure machines measure pulse rate as well as blood pressure. This is useful in order to make a direct correlation between the two parameters during blood pressure measurement when looking for signs of shock. It must be remembered that the measurement will pick up only the peripheral pulses and may not reflect the heart rate: the heart rate will only be truly measured on an ECG tracing or by listening for apex beats.

Most machines will allow the storage of patient data, such as patient name and hospital number, along with the storage of previous recordings. The ability to recall previous recordings can be useful to the practitioner when assessing trends in the patient's condition. Alarm limits are also useful to give the practitioner instant feedback on deteriorating values and should be set appropriately for each individual.

Trouble-shooting

As a result of the method of measurement, an irregular pulse rate can cause machines to remeasure the blood pressure. If the machine is repeatedly attempting to take the blood pressure without success, it may be necessary to resort to using a sphygmomanometer and stethoscope. It is also important to consider patient comfort in this case.

Common problems related to connecting or positioning the equipment can easily be avoided. One example is the kinking of hoses: in this case, it is necessary to ensure that the hoses are correctly positioned before starting measurement or when the patient adjusts his or her position. Loose connections can result from the initial attachment of the cuff and hoses, causing leaks in the system and a failure of the machinery to obtain readings.

Equipment components, for example those made of rubber, can become worn or perish with poor maintenance or ageing. In addition, most cuffs are manufactured with a 'hook-and-loop' style fastener (e.g.

Velcro), which will influence the life of the cuff, the hook-and-loop system becoming less effective with repeated washing of the cuff and extended use. Cuffs should be replaced if they no longer fasten correctly.

Electrocardiogram

The ECG offers the practitioner several valuable pieces of information. It will provide an accurate depiction of heart rate (rather than just pulse rate), allow the practitioner an early warning of potentially harmful arrhythmias and often show electrical signs of changes to cardiac muscle caused by hypoxia (ST segment changes; see below).

What is measured?

The term commonly used to describe the electrical activity generated that causes a subsequent contraction of cardiac muscle is 'depolarization' of the heart, and the ECG is a record of these electrical impulses as they move through the heart. The ECG representation of electrical impulses can then be used to determine normal and abnormal heart activity. The 12-lead ECG is a standard tool in electrocardiographic diagnosis and is most commonly used as a 'one-off' procedure. As the technique requires 10 separate electrode placements and the associated paraphernalia, it is often not practical for continuous electrocardiographic monitoring even though it is a more thorough measurement of the heart's electrical activity. If, however, the specific diagnosis of myocardial ischaemia is sought, a 12-lead ECG will provide a more thorough picture.

The history of electrocardiography

The method normally chosen for continuous cardiac monitoring involves the placement of three electrodes on the anterior of the chest wall (Singer & Webb, 1998). Willem Einthoven, a Dutch scientist and physiologist, developed the use of modern-day three-lead electrocardiography in the early part of the twentieth century, conducting his research by placing his limbs into buckets of saline and recording the impulses of the heart peripherally. His measurements involved calculating the electrical activity between two poles (bipolar readings), positive and negative. Einthoven's work has come to underpin the measurement and representation of modern electrocardiography.

A diagrammatic representation of his measurement points, Einthoven's triangle, is shown in Figure 5.3, these roughly corresponding to the current

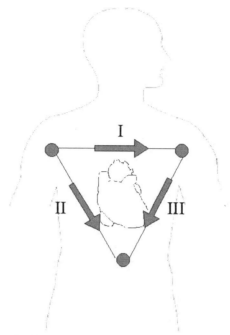

Figure 5.3 Einthoven's triangle.

accepted placement of the chest leads. Also represented are the planes in which the measurements are taken (leads I, II and III) and their corresponding positive and negative poles (the arrows representing the flow from the negative to the positive pole). Measurements of impulses are taken in these planes and then represented by a display in sequence as they happen (Table 5.7). Einthoven also categorized the waves (which he designated P, Q, R, S and T, the middle letters of the alphabet) to depict the electrical sequence of the heart, although he was unaware of their exact meaning.

Table 5.7 ECG leads

Lead I	Right arm (−)	to	Left arm (+)
Lead II	Right arm (−)	to	Left leg (+)
Lead III	Left arm (−)	to	Left leg (+)

Isoelectric line

The flat line, depicted by a lack of impulse readings, is referred to as the isoelectric line. Once the leads have been placed on the chest, any subsequent readings will result from electrical activity. Without other electrical interference, this tracing will represent the electrical impulses generated by the heart, but this cannot always be assumed as muscle can generate electrical impulses and surrounding equipment can also interfere with the isoelectric line. Obtaining a good ECG trace has much to do with minimizing electrical interference from other sources so that the heart's electrical activity can be clearly displayed.

Lead position and placement

The electrodes are normally placed on the right and left sides of the chest just below the clavicles, and at the lower left part of the chest or left upper abdomen (Figure 5.4). Electrodes should not be placed over bony prominences as conduction is better between the intercostal spaces. The areas where the electrodes are to be placed should be clean, dry and free of hair to ensure good adhesion. Effective adhesion can be achieved by preparing the area prior to placement. This includes removing unwanted hair (also improving patient comfort on removal), drying the area (removing perspiration and so on), wiping with an alcohol wipe (to remove oily deposits) and sometimes using a mild exfoliating gel or pad to remove dead skin cells. Modern electrodes consist of an adhesive outer part with a gelatinous centre (conducting jelly) and should be placed such that the adhesive area is pressed into place before the gelatinous centre (so that jelly does not prevent proper adhesion).

After electrode placement, the leads, which are labelled or colour coded, can then be clipped to their corresponding sites. The standard format is as follows: the right arm is labelled RA (red), the left arm LA (yellow), the left leg LL (green) and the right leg RL (black).

The ECG monitor

Once the electrodes and leads have been attached, the tracing obtained from the monitor should be assessed for clarity. Practitioners should ensure that they are getting the most accurate picture they can of the patient's heart rhythm from the display. Most monitors allow the operator to choose the lead position observed. Lead II usually gives the best picture, but it may be necessary to change to leads I or III. In addition, most monitors show the scale with which the electrical activity is displayed, also known as the gain. It may be necessary to increase or decrease this to get a size that allows for a better interpretation of the rhythm.

Monitors have alarm settings that should be set at this stage to ensure that any changes in rhythm are quickly detected. All monitors have heart rate alarms, which should be set closely at approximately the patient's baseline heart rate. Some monitors may have alarms for irregularity of

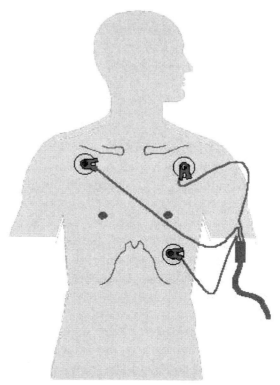

Figure 5.4 ECG electrode placement.

heart rate, which is a good way of detecting such changes. More sophisticated systems are available to detect change in the ST segment and calculate ST elevation or depression. This can highlight any changes caused by hypoxaemia, but the facility is not available in most monitoring systems.

Normal cardiac cycle

The P, Q, R, S and T waves (Figure 5.5) represent the normal cardiac cycle on the ECG tracing. The shape and depth of the deflections will alter depending on which view of the heart is being measured. This representation will roughly equate with the views seen in leads I, II, and III, but the practitioner will need experience of looking at many normal traces.

The P wave represents depolarization of the atria and their subsequent contraction. The QRS complex represents the depolarization of the ventricles and their subsequent contraction, whereas the T wave

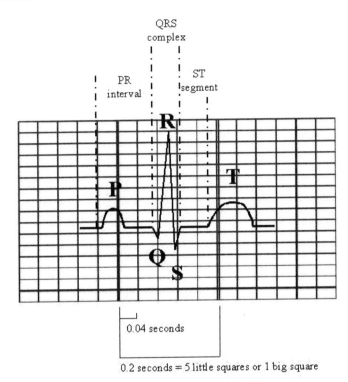

Figure 5.5 The normal cardiac cycle as represented on an ECG.

represents the repolarization phase during which the muscle is at rest and becoming ready for the next depolarization.

The normal time limits for each phase of the cycle are also represented in Figure 5.5; these can be measured by obtaining a rhythm strip (printed on graph paper) and using the grid to calculate them (counting the small squares in between). Widening of the PR interval (to more than 0.2 seconds) or the QRS complex (to more than 0.12 seconds) may indicate altered conduction or conduction through alternate pathways. Elevation or depression of the ST segment may indicate hypoxic or ischaemic changes within the heart (see below).

Common dysrhythmias recognition and significance

Details of these can be found in Rainbow (1989).

Sinus bradycardia

This is a series of impulses generated from the sinoatrial node and therefore possesses all the elements of the PQRST complex. The rate of the impulse will be less than 60 beats per minute. This rhythm can be normal in young, healthy, athletic adults or can be induced by certain medications. In this instance, the rhythm is usually insignificant, but if there is a reason to suspect that there has been a recent change to sinus bradycardia, an underlying pathology should be suspected. It is possible for other serious arrhythmias to develop from sinus bradycardia, particularly if it is a symptom of myocardial infarction. Rhythm strip 1 shows bradycardia at a rate of 40 beats per minute.

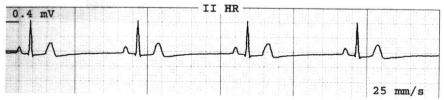

Rhythm strip 1 Bradycardia.

Sinus tachycardia

As with sinus bradycardia, this impulse is generated in the sinoatrial node, but the rate will exceed 100 beats per minute. The rhythm will be regular and the complexes normally shaped. This condition is normal as part of the body's flight or fight mechanism, and the heart rate will usually increase to this level with exertion, anxiety or pain. There can also be underlying pathological causes such as haemorrhage, hypoxia, congestive cardiac failure, left ventricular failure or an overdosage of certain cardiac stimulating drugs. A sustained sinus tachycardia of over 140 beats per minute should be closely monitored as the resulting reduction in ventricular filling time can place a strain on the heart and have a detrimental effect on coronary perfusion. Rhythm strip 2 shows sinus rhythm (80 beats per minute) developing into sinus tachycardia (160 beats per minute).

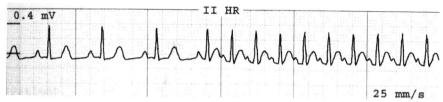

Rhythm strip 2 Sinus rhythm developing into sinus tachycardia.

Sinus arrhythmia

This rhythm has a normal rate of 60–100 beats per minute and normal PQRST complexes. It is common in the young and is linked with respiratory rate. On inspiration and expiration, the vagus nerve (and therefore its influence on the sinoatrial node) is affected, its impulses being speeded up and slowed down respectively. The resulting rhythm is an irregular heart rate with normal PQRST complexes (Rhythm strip 3). This is an asymptomatic rhythm and requires no treatment.

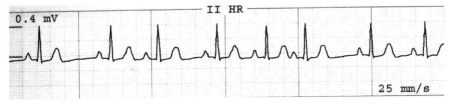

Rhythm strip 3 Sinus arrhythmia.

Atrial extrasystoles

These impulses originate outside the sinoatrial node, the P wave therefore usually being abnormally shaped. They have a narrow QRS complex that appears normal. After the escape beat, there is a pause on the trace, referred to as a compensatory pause. Rhythm strip 4 shows an atrial extrasystole with a P wave of normal shape occurring shortly after a series of normal sinus beats. These beats can be a normal phenomenon but may also indicate an excitable atrium prior to pathological conditions such as atrial fibrillation. Atrial extrasystoles raise concern if they are very frequent and compromise arterial blood pressure.

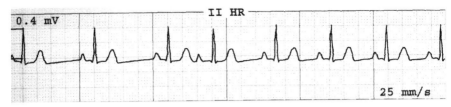

Rhythm strip 4 Atrial extrasystole.

Ventricular extrasystoles

These impulses originate in the ventricle and follow a pathway different from that of normal ventricular beats. The complexes do not therefore have a normal shape and often possess very different deflections from normal. They have a wide QRS complex of abnormal shape and no identifiable P wave activity. The T wave is also commonly abnormal or inverted. The dysrhythmia may take various forms: random beats, alternation between normal beats (bigeminy), the waveform appearing on top of the preceding T wave (the R-on-T phenomenon, which is potentially very harmful), multifocal (with a different shape each time) or consecutive (in a row). The frequency of the ectopic beats is important, because if it is high it may indicate an excitable ventricle and herald potentially fatal arrhythmias. R-on-T ventricular extrasystoles may precipitate ventricular fibrillation since the ventricle is vulnerable at this stage (repolarization). Rhythm strip 5 shows the end of a ventricular extrasystole, followed by two further ventricular extrasystoles.

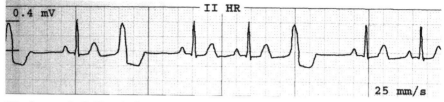

Rhythm strip 5 Ventricular extrasystole.

Atrial flutter

With this arrhythmia, the atrium is sending impulses at a rate of 250–350 beats per minute, the resulting pattern of the baseline being described as 'sawtooth'. As the atrioventricular node cannot accept these impulses at the speed at which it receives them, the ventricular rate is much slower. This is a form of block, the ventricle commonly accepting 1 out of 2 (a 2:1 block with a ventricular rate of 150 beats per minute), 1 out of 3 (a 3:1 block, the ventricular rate being 100 beats per minute) or 1 out of 4 (the 4:1 block ventricular rate being 75 beats per minute). The rate is usually regular but may become irregular if the atrioventricular block changes. This block occasionally fluctuates, a 2:1 block becoming a 3:1 block and then a 4:1 block, or any variation of the three occurring.

In this rhythm the QRS complex is normal (rather than broad) as conduction in the ventricle follows the normal pathway. Rhythm strip 6 shows atrial flutter with varying block; note the baseline. This rhythm can become potentially life-threatening, and treatment will depend on the ventricular rate (if high) and whether there is cardiovascular compromise.

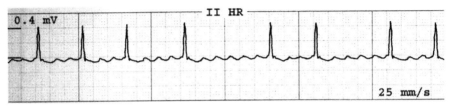

Rhythm strip 6 Atrial flutter.

Atrial fibrillation

Atrial fibrillation is described as an irregularly irregular rhythm (with no definable pattern) and is characterized by irregular QRS impulses without discernible P waves. The atrium is sending off a multitude of impulses and is described as looking like a bag of worms. Some of the impulses will make their way through the atrioventricular node and go on to produce a QRS complex, but this is rather a hit-and-miss affair. The resulting ventricular activity will depend on how many impulses are received by the atrioventricular node, which varies greatly. The QRS complex is normal, but the baseline is described as wavy or erratic. With atrial fibrillation, the atria are ineffective and the volume of blood being injected to the ventricles is reduced.

Atrial fibrillation can be asymptomatic, but with a high ventricular rate and underlying disease, the patient's blood pressure may become compromised. In this case, treatment may be required to slow down the ventricular response. Rhythm strip 7 shows atrial fibrillation; note the irregularity of the QRS rate and the wiggly baseline.

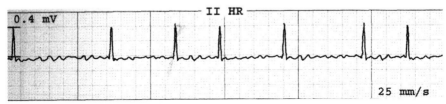

Rhythm strip 7 Atrial fibrillation.

Life-threatening dysrhythmias recognition and significance

All of these dysrhythmias (Rainbow, 1989) will demand emergency intervention, and most will require the instigation of advanced life support techniques.

Ventricular tachycardia

This rhythm is generated from within the ventricle from one or more foci and has a rate of 140–220 beats per minute. The P waves are not visible as they are swamped by the QRS complexes, which are wide and bizarre in shape. Ventricular tachycardia can arise spontaneously but often is preceded by runs (salvos) of ventricular ectopic beats. Recognizing increasing ventricular activity can alert the practitioner to the occurrence of this potentially life-threatening rhythm. Treatment will depend on blood pressure and the patient's level of consciousness, but sustained ventricular tachycardia must be treated. Rhythm strip 8 shows ventricular tachycardia; note the broad QRS complexes.

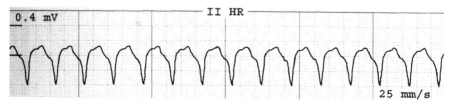

Rhythm strip 8 Ventricular tachycardia.

Ventricular fibrillation

The rhythm in ventricular fibrillation is generated by many sources within the ventricle and is classified as fine or coarse. Coarse ventricular fibrillation responds better to treatment and is usually the precursor of fine ventricular fibrillation. This latter rhythm has no life-sustaining cardiac output and needs advanced life support to be initiated immediately (Resuscitation Council, 2000). Rhythm strip 9 shows coarse ventricular fibrillation.

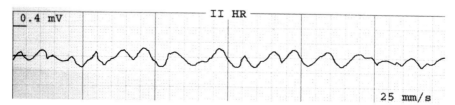

Rhythm strip 9 Ventricular fibrillation.

Asystole

Asystole is the complete absence of electrical activity in the heart and is represented by a flat line. It is sometimes useful to increase the gain on the ECG to rule out fine ventricular fibrillation as this will alter treatment. The patient will have no cardiac output, and advanced life support must be instigated immediately.

ST segment elevation and depression

Alterations of the ST segment may be indicative of ischaemic or hypoxic changes in the cardiac muscle, although, as previously stated, a more complete picture of ischaemic or hypoxic changes will be obtained from a 12-lead ECG. The severity or extent of the damage is difficult to assess using this method, and there is limited evidence in this field that a direct correlation can be found (Moons et al., 1999). In the endoscopy suite, a recognition of ST segment changes during continual monitoring can alert the practitioner to potentially harmful changes and speed up intervention to prevent these. It is important to be aware of how the ST segment might alter and what this might infer. Figure 5.6 is a set of diagrammatic representations of changes that may occur to the ST segment and their probable causes. Further reading is recommended for those interested in studying the significance of these changes in detail.

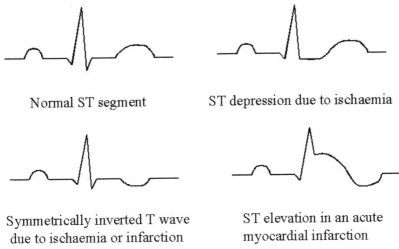

Normal ST segment   ST depression due to ischaemia

Symmetrically inverted T wave   ST elevation in an acute
due to ischaemia or infarction   myocardial infarction

Figure 5.6 ST segment changes.

Conclusion

This chapter has covered the clinical and mechanical methods of continuous monitoring before and during endoscopic procedures under sedation, but monitoring must continue into the recovery period and up until discharge. The major emphasis of this chapter is that mechanical means of monitoring are not simply recording devices to be placed on fingers, arms or chests. The decision to use such devices should arise from clinical judgement, and this should also provide the framework within which the readings are analysed. It is the practitioner's experience and the knowledge level that make for thorough and effective monitoring.

A selection of dysrhythmias were displayed in this chapter, but this is only a selection and will not reflect every rhythm seen on an ECG. Experience in interpretating ECGs is essential before the practitioner can assess what is and what is not important. Further reading will improve the practitioner's understanding of ECG interpretation.

Throughout the chapter, the risks associated with sedation and endoscopic procedures have been outlined, the main ones being associated with respiratory and cardiovascular complications. A knowledge of advanced life support techniques is essential within this environment as complications can ultimately lead to cardiorespiratory arrest. Prevention is, however, better than cure, and effective monitoring should aim for the early recognition of complications.

References

British Society of Gastroenterology (1991) Endoscopy Section Committee Working Party: recommendations for standards of sedation and patient monitoring during gastrointestinal endoscopy. Gut 32: 823–7.

British Society of Gastroenterology (1995) Clinical Guidelines: Gastro-intestinal Endoscopy in General Practice. London: BSG.

Charlton JE (1995) Monitoring and supplemental oxygen during endoscopy. British Medical Journal 310: 886–7.

Hanning CD, Alexander-Williams JM (1995) Fortnightly review: Pulse oximetry: a practical review. British Medical Journal 311: 367–70.

Kost M (1998) Manual of Conscious Sedation. Philadelphia: WB Saunders.

Moons K, Klootwijk P, Meij S et al. (1999) Continuous ST-segment monitoring associated with infarct size and left ventricular function in the GUSTO-I trial. American Heart Journal 138(3): 525–32.

Moyle JTB, Hahn CEW, Adams AP (1994) Pulse Oximetry. Principles and Practice Series. London: BMJ Publishing Group.

Owen A (1992) Pocket Guide to Critical Care Monitoring. St Louis: Mosby-Year Book.

Quine MA, Bell GD, McCloy RF, Charlton JE, Devlin HB, Hopkins A (1995) Prospective audit of upper gastrointestinal endoscopy in two regions of England: safety, staffing, and selection methods. Gut 36: 462–7.

Rainbow C (1989) Monitoring the Critically Ill Patient. Oxford: Heinemann Nursing.

Reed MWR, Reilly CS (1995) Hypoxia during endoscopy also occurs in unsedated patients. British Medical Journal 311: 453.

Resuscitation Council (2000) ALS Course Provider Manual, 4th edn. London: Resuscitation Council.

Royal College of Surgeons of England (1993) Report of the Working Party on Guidelines for Sedation by Non-anaesthetists. London: Commission on the Provision of Surgical Services.

Shoemaker WC, Ayres SM, Grenvik A, Holbrook PR (2000) Textbook of Critical Care, 4th edn. Philadelphia: WB Saunders.

Singer M, Webb A (1998) Oxford Handbook of Critical Care. New York: Oxford University Press.
Society of American Gastrointestinal Endoscopic Surgeons (1996) Guidelines for Office Endoscopic Services. www.sages.org/sgpub9.html
Stephenson A (1998) A Textbook of General Practice. London: Arnold.
Swash M (1995) Hutchinson's Clinical Methods, 20th edn. London: WB Saunders.

Further reading

Appadurai IA, Delicta RJ, Carey PD (1995) Monitoring during endoscopy. British Medical Journal 311: 452.
Bell GD (1991) Monitoring and safety in endoscopy. Baillière's Clinical Gastroenterology 5(1): 79–98.
Cotton P, Williams C (1996) Practical Gastrointestinal Endoscopy, 4th edn. Oxford: Blackwell Scientific.
Hampton JR (1986) The ECG in Practice. Edinburgh: Churchill Livingstone.
Honeybourne D, Neumann CS (1997) An audit of bronchoscopy practice in the United Kingdom: a survey of adherence to national guidelines. Thorax 52: 709–13.
Kidwell JE (1991) Nursing care for the patient receiving conscious sedation during gastrointestinal endoscopic procedures. Society of Gastroenterology Nurses and Associates (Winter): 134–9.
Kimmey MB, Al-Kawas FH, Gannan RM et al. (1995) Technology assessment status evaluation: monitoring equipment for endoscopy. American Society for Gastrointestinal Endoscopy 42(6): 615–17.
Peri V, Gatto G, Amuso M, Traina M (1995) Italian data support upper gastrointestinal endoscopy without sedation. British Medical Journal 311: 453.
Woodrow P (1999) Pulse oximetry. Nursing Standard 13(42): 42–6.

CHAPTER 6

Assessment of conscious sedation levels

SHEILA MAIR

Gastrointestinal endoscopy is an increasingly common examination used for both diagnosis and therapy. Patients attending an endoscopy unit for an examination, usually as outpatients, are inevitably nervous and apprehensive. For many, it will be their first experience of hospital, and they may, as a result of extreme anxiety, express a wish to be unconscious during the examination. The endoscopist, on the other hand, prefers a patient who is co-operative and relaxed: patient co-operation is important in order to facilitate the procedure and any necessary interventions. Patients may also require more than one examination and may discuss their experience with other potential patients. These factors alone make it important that the experience is made as tolerable and as stress free as possible. One way to do this is to use the technique of conscious sedation.

For nurse practitioners involved in the administration of conscious sedation, there are several basic questions to consider. First, what is meant by the term 'conscious sedation'? Second, how do you know whether a patient is adequately sedated? Third, is it possible to measure just how sedated a patient is and is there indeed any merit in so doing? Finally, and just as importantly, what should the nurse do if the sedation is inadequate?

What is conscious sedation?

The Royal College of Surgeons (1993) has defined conscious sedation as:

> a technique in which the use of a drug or drugs produces a state of depression of the central nervous system enabling treatment to be carried out, but during which communication is maintained such that the patient will respond to command throughout the period of sedation.

Patients will ideally also have an increased tolerance to pain. In addition, a degree of amnesia for the event should make the examination more acceptable to patients and reduce their anxiety about any future examinations. Pearson (1991) emphasizes that what is desired is a patient who is relaxed and conscious and who has little recollection of the procedure.

Booth (1996) describes a continuum along which consciousness gradually progresses through sedation to unconsciousness, anaesthesia, coma and eventually death. Conscious sedation becomes general anaesthesia if there is a loss of contact with the patient (Royal College of Surgeons of England, 1993). The practitioner who administers sedation to such a degree that the patient loses consciousness is therefore inducing anaesthesia and practising as an anaesthetist.

How do you know whether the patient is adequately sedated?

Mr Brown is undergoing a flexible sigmoidoscopy carried out under intravenous sedation with midazolam. He is lying comfortably on his left side and is able to turn on to his back when asked to do so by the endoscopist. During the examination, he lies dozing, opening his eyes every now and then when the nurse speaks to him. Mr Brown's pulse rate and oxygen saturation have hardly changed since the start of the examination, and he is surprised to be told that the examination has been completed. Mr Brown and the nurse would both consider that sedation was adequate. Mr Brown showed no signs of anxiety, did not complain of pain, was unaware of time passing but nevertheless remained conscious and cooperative throughout.

A nurse may intuitively believe that the level of sedation is correct. The patient lies quietly relaxed, is conscious but not anxious, and responds to verbal stimuli but otherwise may respond only to noxious stimuli. The patient is able to maintain his or her own airway and shows minimal changes in vital signs, blood pressure, heart rate and rhythm, as well as oxygen saturation. At the end of such an episode, the nurse will probably state that the patient tolerated the procedure well.

Such a comment, however, does little to describe to anyone else the patient's actual demeanour. 'Tolerate' often implies a state of putting up with something or enduring it. Does this mean that the patient lay with white knuckles holding on to the sides of the trolley? Did the patient hold his breath for the best, or worst, part of the examination? Did the patient lie quietly because he was unconscious and totally unaware of what was going on around him? It would be helpful to have some means of describing in more detail how patients cope with the examination and respond to the sedation.

A sedation scale or score can provide a guide to level of sedation desired and whether the aims of sedation have been met. The Association of Operating Room Nurses (AORN, 1997) states that the objectives for the patient receiving conscious sedation include the maintenance of consciousness while elevating the pain threshold. There should also be an alteration in mood, a decrease in anxiety level and a minimal variation in vital signs. Ideally, there should also be some degree of amnesia and finally a quick return to the normal activities of daily living. Any measurement will involve the patient being observed and is a first step in ensuring patient comfort and safety. So the patient undergoing endoscopy will be relaxed and co-operative, will have little disturbance of vital signs and will possess some degree of amnesia of the event.

Why measure conscious sedation level?

The nurse's primary concern is with the patient's well-being, so there needs to be some system of measuring and documenting this. Patients' well-being includes how comfortable they are, changes in their vital signs and how they are tolerating the examination. Nurses already assess and plan care and evaluate the outcome of any intervention, all these stages being documented in care plans and nursing notes. It would therefore seem logical that, having assessed the patient as being anxious and having administered sedation, the endoscopist should be able to measure the effect of this intervention, just as pain relief is measured after analgesia is given. Part of the patient's comfort and well-being relates to the level of conscious sedation, so a measure of sedation can therefore be part of the general measurements of patient comfort. In this way, assessing the level of consciousness, using a measurement tool to ensure accuracy, can be seen as part of nursing care.

Another reason for assessing conscious sedation is that sedation techniques carry risks. The drugs most commonly used are benzodiazepines, which have side effects. Roche (1992) list adverse reactions and side effects including cardiovascular changes, for example a decrease in mean arterial pressure, cardiac output and stroke volume, as well as respiratory depression and respiratory arrest. Benjamin (1996) describes adverse effects associated with drug administration, including oversedation, overmedication, cardiac arrhythmias and respiratory insufficiency. Anaphylaxis is also a possible complication. It has been suggested that 50% of all cases of morbidity and 60% of those of mortality occurring with upper gastrointestinal endoscopy are related to hypoxaemia caused by conscious sedation (Froehlich et al., 1995).

Pearson (1991) records the incidence of respiratory depression as being 0.3% for benzodiazepines. The respiratory effects of the benzodiazepines may result partly from their depressant effect on the CNS and partly from their muscle relaxant effect (Reid, 1997). When sedative doses are used, there is a drop in tidal volume, which is usually compensated for by an increase in respiratory rate. If larger doses are used, however, respiratory effects can vary from a reduced minute volume to apnoea (Dundee et al., 1991). The risk is also increased when these are used in combination with other drugs, including analgesics such as pethidine.

The use of an appropriate scale with continuous monitoring of the level of sedation is the first step in identifying, for example, early signs of respiratory depression. If measurements of conscious sedation level are made frequently, any decrease in response will be noted early. A decrease in responsiveness may precede changes in oxygen saturation as an indicator of an increasing depth of sedation. Measuring the level of sedation can therefore be seen as a means of avoiding giving excessive doses of sedation and of rectifying the situation promptly if this inadvertently occurs.

The relationship between dose and effect is not straightforward as individuals, especially children, the elderly and those who are frail, vary in their response to drugs. Undersedation may be more easily detected than oversedation as the patient who is undersedated is likely to have more overt symptoms. The patient who is restless, complaining of discomfort and unco-operative is impossible to ignore whilst the patient who is lying quietly is easily overlooked.

The documentation of level of consciousness should allow future episodes to be managed well, which is vitally important as a well-managed sedation experience results in the patient being willing to attend in the future. In addition, with an increasing number of people being referred for diagnostic and screening examinations, the patients of today will influence those of tomorrow. The fact that the sedation experience is, relatively speaking, short and may affect whether the patient comes for further examinations makes it particularly important to get it right first time.

An understanding of how a previous sedation episode was managed can help in planning subsequent sessions. Furthermore, well-managed sedation allows a complete examination to be carried out, particularly in an otherwise overanxious or unco-operative patient: if the sedation is inadequate, a complete examination may be impossible. On the other hand, a successful examination may be pointless if the patient suffers as a result of oversedation.

A tool that can be used to assess sedation level can and should be used as a teaching aid. This ensures that all staff are aware of the scale itself, the parameters being measured and the importance of each of those parameters. Safety and quality of care can be threatened if there is a misunderstanding of the aims for conscious sedation. If the nurse perceives that the aim of sedation is for the patient to lie motionless for the duration of the examination, the amount of sedation required to reach that desired state may be such that the patient will suffer from respiratory depression or worse.

Finally, in an age of increasing litigation, documentation is important to protect the nurse – if it is not documented, it is not done. Moreover, documentation can improve communication between staff and therefore improves continuity of care. It also allows a quality of care measurement as actual outcomes can be compared with expected outcomes. Accurate documentation is good risk management, and good risk management is good patient care.

In order to monitor the level of sedation, the nurse must be able to identify what comprises an optimal conscious sedation episode and then find some way of measuring and documenting this.

How can the level of conscious sedation be measured?

Observing the pulse rate, blood pressure and oxygen saturation will provide an indication of the patient's clinical condition. Pulse oximetry will alert the nurse to the presence of hypoxaemia and also measure heart rate, but oximetry measures only oxygen saturation rather than the adequacy of ventilation. Monitoring oxygen saturation may therefore indicate the effect that the sedation has on the patient's saturation level but not how effective the sedation is. Measures of haemodynamic variables such as pulse, blood pressure and pulse oximetry data thus measure clinical status rather than level of sedation. Nor is the amount of the drug administered necessarily an indication of the level of consciousness of the patient. Patients respond differently to drugs and not necessarily in a way that can be predicted. A little old lady can sometimes require as much sedation as a young, fit, healthy man.

Level of consciousness is a difficult variable to measure. Consciousness has been described as having two parts to it: arousal or wakefulness, and cognition (Shah, 1999). It is obvious when a patient is deeply unconscious as there is no response to painful stimuli. By the same token, it is easy to establish that a patient is totally conscious, but the grades in between are more difficult to establish (when, for example, does light sedation become deep sedation?) and are open to subjective opinion. In conscious sedation, the patient should have some degree of wakefulness and should be able to respond appropriately to verbal commands. When nurses are assessing conscious sedation, they are, however, interested not only in the level of consciousness, but also in whether the aims of conscious sedation have been met. There is currently therefore no one variable that, when measured, will indicate the level of conscious sedation. Instead, the measurement of conscious sedation involves assessing a set of observations taken together. Moreover, these observations rely on a subjective interpretation of the patient's reaction to the sedation. What is required is a scale that describes, as objectively as possible, the behavioural and physiological reactions to sedation (Clark, 1994). This can then formalize the nurse's observations and provide a written record for future use.

What should a tool measure and what qualities should it have?

It is suggested that a tool needs to have both reliability and validity. Reliability refers to the assessment tool's ability consistently to measure the given attribute. The tool will, when used on several occasions in the same given circumstances, produce the same measurement. A thermometer could be said to have good reliability if it consistently measured boiling water at 100°C; it would be unreliable if it did otherwise. A conscious sedation tool must be able to be used by different people on the same patient and still produce the same score, an attibute known as interrater reliability.

Validity is the degree to which the tool measures what it is supposed to be measuring. Although a tool can be reliable without being valid, it cannot be valid unless it is also reliable. That is, a tape measure can reliably measure distance but it is not a valid tool for the measurement of temperature. A tool to measure the level of conscious sedation therefore needs not only to be reliable, but also to measure the level of conscious sedation rather than some other attribute. In this context, it should measure whether the aims of conscious sedation have been achieved. For a fuller discussion of validity, the reader is referred to a standard textbook on research, for example Polit and Hungler (1993).

For practical purposes, any scale needs to be user friendly. If the scale is to be used as a matter of routine, it should be easy to chart and not involve too much extra work. The documentation should also fit easily into the existing framework, be easy to understand and whenever possible avoid subjective descriptions. From the patient's point of view, it needs to be non- or minimally invasive and cause no discomfort.

The ideal tool is currently not yet available, but tools do exist that attempt to measure sedation level. Scales that measure levels of consciousness have been in existence for some time now, one of the best known being the Glasgow coma scale. This was developed in 1974 for use with patients with neurological problems (Teasdale and Jennett, 1974); it provides an easy means of assessing level of consciousness and also has high interrater reliability. It was, however, not designed for use with patients in whom the conscious level is deliberately being altered and therefore does not address the aims of conscious sedation. As a result, a tool such as this is not refined enough for the purposes of measuring sedation and is not therefore valid.

Other scales have been designed with the sedated patient in mind. The Ramsay level of sedation scale (Ramsay et al., 1974) was designed for patients in intensive care receiving sedation and grades sedation on a scale from 1 to 6, 1 denoting a patient who is anxious, agitated or restless, and 6 a patient who is non-responsive. This scale is simple to use but on its own tells very little about how the patient coped with the examination; nor are the aims of conscious sedation addressed.

Another scale, which has been widely used, is the Aldrete scale (Table 6.1) (Aldrete and Kroulik, 1970). This was designed for use in the theatre recovery area and aims to measure the patient's progress on recovery from anaesthesia. Five parameters are measured: activity, respiration, circulation, consciousness and oxygenation. This tool therefore looks at the patient in more detail.

This modified version of the scale has now been expanded to address the needs of patients undergoing day surgery. The expanded version includes scoring for wound dressing, pain, ambulation, fasting/feeding and urine output. Although not all of these parameters are required for endoscopy patients, the scale could perhaps be used where endoscopy and day surgery patients are cared for in the same area. As with previous scales, this was not designed for the assessment of conscious sedation, but given that conscious sedation is a point on a continuum from consciousness at

Table 6.1 Aldrete scale

		Admission	5 min	15 min	30 min	45 min	60 min	discharge
Able to move four extremities voluntarily or on command	2	Activity						
Able to move two extremities voluntarily or on command	1							
Unable to move extremities voluntarily or on command	0							
Able to breathe deeply and cough freely	2	Respiratory						
Dyspnoea or limited breathing	1							
Apnoeic	0							
BP + 20% of preanaesthetic level	2	Circulation						
BP + 20–49% of preanaesthetic level	1							
BP + 50% of preanaesthetic level	0							
Fully awake	2	Consciousness						
Arousable on calling	1							
Not responding	0							
Able to maintain oxygen saturation 92% on room air	2	Oxygen saturation						
Needs oxygen inhalation to maintain oxygen saturation 90%	1							
Oxygen saturation <90% even with oxygen supplementation	0							
		Totals						

one end through to anaesthesia and coma at the other, it could be argued that this is a suitable scale. Furthermore, there are certain advantages in using only one scale in any one area. Nursing staff become familiar with the scale and quick at scoring, and there is less opportunity for confusion if only one scale is used.

What little research there is into conscious sedation scoring has on the whole been carried out in order to develop scales for use with critically ill patients. The question then arises of whether a tool designed for use with one patient population can be accurately employed with another. Clark (1994), who developed a tool for use in the endoscopy setting, has addressed this problem (Table 6.2). Using the aims of conscious sedation as laid out by the AORN, she describes five parameters to be assessed: emotional affect, level of consciousness, physical reaction to discomfort or pain, variation in vital signs and degree of amnesia. The scale recognizes three degrees of sedation: optimal sedation, oversedation and undersedation. The scoring system is such that it indicates only whether sedation is optimal or suboptimal rather than whether the direction is under- or oversedation. Objectivity has been addressed by specifying percentiles when appropriate. Optimal sedation scores between 8 and 10.

The validity and reliability of this tool have been tested, and it has been shown that it requires some further refinement. Despite not being perfect, this tool goes, however, a long way to providing an accurate description of patient response to intravenous conscious sedation.

Table 6.2 Clark conscious sedation scale

Parameter (circle one)	Grade		
	0	1	2
Emotional affect 0 1 2	1. Flat affect 2. Does not respond to commands or stimuli	1. Anxious or uneasy (50%) 2. Does not respond to commands appropriately	1. Quiescent, tranquil (75%) 2. Responds to commands appropriately
Level of consciousness 0 1 2	1. Unarousable/stuporous 2. Protective reflexes absent	1. Intermittent arousal or awake/aware 2. Protective reflexes present	1. Drowsy or asleep, easily rousable 2. Protective reflexes present
Physical reaction to discomfort or pain 0 1 2	1. Flaccid/non-responsive 2. No exhibition or complaint of discomfort or pain	1. Restless and/or resistive 2. Vocalization throughout majority of procedure (50%)	1. Generally at ease/rest 2. May occasionally exhibit symptoms or vocalize to complain of discomfort or pain
Variation in vital signs 0 1 2	1. Respiratory depression and/or decrease in cardiovascular function 2. Intervention necessary	1. No beneficial change in respiratory or cardiovascular function	1. Therapeutic alteration in respiratory/cardio-vascular function 2. No intervention necessary
Degree of amnesia 0 1 2	1. Total amnesia (secondary to stuporous condition and loss of protective reflexes)	1. Recall of 75–100% of procedure	1. Minimal (%) recall or total amnesia

Whichever scale is used, there will be an opportunity for nurses to observe the patient and document these observations, but scales and scores are meaningless if nurses do not act on their findings. It therefore goes without saying that merely documenting a score is not enough: any score other than an optimal score requires the nurse to take action.

What if sedation is inadequate?

A system of scoring may go a long way to helping to achieve the ideal episode of sedation, but the mere fact that conscious sedation can be scored does not mean that every sedation episode will be perfect. It is sometimes difficult to sedate the patient adequately without then running the risk of inducing anaesthesia because of the large dose of the drug required. On other occasions, the sedation appears to have an almost paradoxical effect on the patient, who then becomes more restless and agitated. On yet other occasions, the procedure lasts longer than anticipated and the initial dose of sedation is no longer adequate but additional sedation is contraindicated.

Take the example of Mr Green, who has been adequately sedated for his sigmoidoscopy but biopsies need to be taken. The examination has lasted more than 20 minutes because of difficulty negotiating the rectosigmoid junction and the presence of multiple diverticula. Mr Green, whose pulse rate and oxygen saturation have all remained within normal limits for him, has now become uncomfortable and distressed. He asks that the examination be terminated. What should the nurse do to help Mr Green?

The scope can be withdrawn, in which case the patient has had an incomplete examination, biopsies have not been obtained and he may require another examination about which he is unlikely to be enthusiastic given that he found the first one distressing. The examination could continue, with or without more sedation, in which case the endoscopist could be accused of assault as the patient has withdrawn consent for the procedure. Furthermore, if the patient is unco-operative or very restless and distressed, the endoscopist runs the added risk of harming the patient, including the risk of perforation of the bowel. Pain during an endoscopic examination may be an indication that there is damage, or the potential for damage, to the bowel or mesentery and should always be investigated.

What is the nurse's role in this case? The nurse endoscopist might be inclined to try to finish the examination, knowing that it would save a repeat visit, but this would have to be balanced by the need to perform the examination safely. As the patient's advocate, however, the nurse may decide to halt the examination. If the nurse stops the examination and the patient then cannot remember asking for this, he will probably not be too apprehensive about attending for a second examination on the basis that the first one was, for him, unremarkable. If, however, the patient does remember the examination, the fact that his request to stop the examination was acceded to should reaffirm that he is in control.

From the late 1980s, one of the nurse's important roles has been to act as an advocate for the patient. There has been some debate about whether nurses have always acted as patients' advocates or whether this is a new role development resulting from the increasing demand for and expectation of patients' rights. This role has not been made explicit; indeed, the *Code of Professional Conduct* (UKCC, 1992) merely implies advocacy. The role of the nurse as patient's advocate is a difficult one at any time. An advocate is, according to the *Oxford Dictionary*, one who pleads for another. The Royal College of Nursing (1992) meanwhile has defined advocacy as 'a process of acting for, or on behalf of someone who is unable to do so for themselves'.

There are several reasons why a patient may need an advocate. It has been suggested that the imbalance of power between the patient and the medical or healthcare staff is the prime reason. This imbalance may arise from a patient's relative lack of knowledge or when patients are vulnerable, for example when their health is compromised or when they are in unfamiliar surroundings.

The nurse's role as the patient's advocate is fraught with difficulties. Before acting in this way, there must be some invitation from the patient to do so: acting as the patient's advocate when the patient does not wish it cannot be seen as true advocacy. The nurse cannot decide what is in the interests of the patient – only the patient can do this. The patient requires information in order to make a decision, which the nurse should then support. In the context of nursing, this usually requires the nurse to ensure that patients have enough information in order to make a decision about their care. The nurse therefore has to decide how much information, and of what depth, is required, so the nurse still has power. Furthermore, some patients do not want to make decisions about their care and prefer the healthcare professional to make the decisions for them. In such circumstances, it is difficult for the nurse to act as the patient's advocate: there is no way of knowing what the patient might want if he is unwilling to discuss the examination with the nurse in the first place.

The role of the nurse as advocate has been thought of as being important with particular reference to the imbalance of power between patient and doctor. It can, however, just as easily reflect an imbalance between nurse and patient, particularly when the nurse is taking on a role that is normally associated with the medical profession, although patients may perceive a smaller power imbalance between nurse and patient than between doctor and patient.

So where does this leave the patient? The nurse who is normally the advocate is now performing the examination. Can the nurse fulfil both roles? The medical profession face this dilemma every day but have nurses to help patients in their decision-making. Does this mean that the nurse as endoscopist relinquishes the role of advocate to the endoscopy nurse?

There is no clear answer, but it may be better to think of the nurse as helping to empower the patient. This means that patients will still speak out for themselves but nurses will make it easier for them to do so. This may mean drawing the endoscopist's attention to the fact that the patient wishes to speak or halt the examination.

Alternative strategies

When sedation is inadequate, it is still possible to continue the examination by using alternative techniques, but for these to be effective the patient must trust the nurse. Creating an atmosphere of honesty and mutual respect best fosters this trust. Open communication should be encouraged from the outset. Patients should be able to feel in control or have some say in when they relinquish that control. Those having a gastric endoscopy may be asked to raise their hand if they would like the examination to be stopped at any stage. The patient undergoing flexible sigmoidoscopy must be encouraged to tell the endoscopist if the examination is painful. If the nurse states that the examination will be halted if it becomes uncomfortable, he or she must be prepared to do this as soon as the patient indicates.

McCaffery (1983) suggested that increased anxiety leads to an increased perception of pain. Anxiety can lead not only to an increased focus on the pain, but also increased muscle tension, which can in itself cause an increase in pain. A patient's pain or anxiety should not be dismissed or trivialized but assessed and dealt with appropriately. For some patients, this may mean the administration of analgesia, for others a further dose of sedation. Still others will require support and encouragement to get them through a short but uncomfortable stage of the examination. Sedation is sometimes suboptimal, and where more sedation is contraindicated or undesirable, the nurse must rely on alternative techniques to ease the patient's discomfort.

Clear explanations of what to expect during the procedure, with sensory as well as procedural information, will help to prepare patients. If patients realize that it is normal to be aware of what is going on around them from time to time during the examination, they are less likely to panic than if they are expecting to be completely anaesthetized and unaware of anything.

Various techniques may help a patient through difficult stages of the examination. Sometimes just stopping for a minute to allow the patient gain control can help. An explanation of the reason for the discomfort, such as abdominal cramp, may help to reduce anxiety. Some patients may find the feeling of wanting to pass wind, or the senstation that their bowels are about to move, extremely distressing. These patients can be reminded that such feelings are normal and that the cause is the bowel distension caused by the insufflation of air. The endoscopist can help by removing some of the air if it is causing distress.

Slow, gentle breathing can also be of benefit; those who practise yoga and/or forms of relaxation, and women who have attended antenatal classes, can all be encouraged to use their breathing techniques. For others unfamiliar with relaxation techniques, encouraging them to focus on their breathing may act as enough of a distraction to allow the examination to be completed.

Simple distraction can be effective, and the nurse can encourage conversation during an examination of the lower bowel. Some endoscopy units have music playing, which can also be used for distraction purposes. In some cases, watching the examination on the video screen during lower gastrointestinal examinations can keep the patient's mind occupied as well as providing an opportunity for patient education.

Whenever sedation has been inadequate, it is important to spend time with the patient after the examination explaining possible causes of the inadequacy and remedies for any future examinations. Patients need to be assured that the endoscopist was at all times endeavouring to act in their best interests. It may be that the patient had an unrealistic expectation of the sedation. Some patients would like to be totally unaware of the examination, but this would necessitate the administration of a general anaesthetic, which in itself increases risk and requires the services of an anaesthetist and anaesthetic machines. A clear description of the aim of sedation before the examination may avoid some problems, and further discussion afterwards can clarify any misunderstandings about the nature of sedation.

The patient needs to be assured that any future examinations will be managed in such a way as to improve the experience. It may be that the patient's level of anxiety was particularly high to start with, and it may be possible to reduce this by giving a premedication. Scheduling any future examinations for a different time of day may be useful: some patients can control their anxiety for a short time but cannot tolerate waiting until the end of the session. For others, simply being in hospital is a cause of anxiety, and although premedication may be required for these patients, they can also be encouraged to have someone with them who can help them to remain calm. This could be their partner or, in the case of ward patients, their named nurse.

Analgesia may be required for those whose pain has been the prime cause of their inadequate sedation. Patients who normally take analgesics or anti-inflammatory drugs may have gone without them as part of preparing for the examination, and it may be that either these can be taken, an alternative can be given intravenously or the examination can be scheduled for a time when the patient is likely to be more comfortable. Attention should also be paid to any physical problems that are likely to hinder a successful examination: pillows and supports can, for example, be used to support arthritic joints. If the patient feels confident that the nurse is aware of any underlying condition and is able to help, he or she is more likely to be able to relax. Bowel spasm can be a cause of pain and can also make the examination longer or more difficult. This can be reduced by the use of a drug such as hyoscine N-butylbromide.

Even after discussing all possible measures, there will, however, always be some patients for whom the best remedy is an alternative examination, for example a barium enema or barium swallow. Patients should not be made to feel that they have failed but should be reassured that, for them, another examination may be more appropriate. Finally, a general anaesthetic will sometimes be necessary, and the medical staff will need to discuss this with the patient. Whatever the case, the nurse must provide the patient with information and support to undergo any future investigations with the minimum of apprehension.

Summary

The assessment of sedation levels provides:

1. a means of monitoring the effect of sedation on the patient;
2. a tool for quality measurement and risk management;
3. a teaching aid;
4. improved communications;
5. documentation for future sedation episodes.

A good instrument should be valid and reliable, as well as easy and quick to use.

Alternative strategies include:

1. relaxation;
2. distraction;
3. explanation and reassurance.

References

Aldrete JA, Kroulik D (1970) A post-anaesthetic recovery score. Anaesthesia and Analgesia 49: 924–33.

Association of Operating Room Nurses (1997) Recommended practices for managing the patient receiving conscious sedation/analgesia. AORN Journal 65(1): 129–34.

Benjamin SB (1996) Complications of conscious sedation. Gastrointestinal Endoscopy Clinics of North America 6(2): 277–86.

Booth M (1996) Clinical aspects of nurse anesthesia practice: sedation and monitored anesthetic care. Nursing Clinics of North America 31: 667–82.

Clark B (1994) A new approach to assessment and documentation of conscious sedation during endoscopic examinations. Gastroenterology Nursing 16: 199–203.

Dundee JW, Clarke RSJ, McCaughey W (1991) Clinical Anaesthetic Pharmacology. Edinburgh: Churchill Livingstone.

Froehlich F, Schwizer W, Thorens J, Kohler M, Gonvers J-J, Fried M (1995) Conscious sedation for gastroscopy: patient tolerance and cardiorespiratory parameters. Gastroenterology 108(3): 697–704.

McCaffery M (1983) Nursing the Patient in Pain. London: Harper & Row.

Pearson R (1991) The rationale for sedation in endoscopy. In: McCloy R (ed.) Towards Safer Sedation. Roche.

Polit DF, Hungler BP (1993) Essentials of Nursing Research Methods: Appraisal and Utilization. Philadelphia: JB Lippincott.

Ramsay M, Savage T, Simpson B, Goodwin R (1974) Controlled sedation with alphaxalone. British Medical Journal 2: 656–9.

Reid E (1997) Intravenous sedation for short procedures and investigations. Nursing Standard 12(5): 36–8.

Royal College of Nursing (1992) Issues in Nursing and Health: Advocacy and the Nurse. London: RCN.

Royal College of Surgeons of England (1993) Guidelines for Sedation by Non-anaesthetists. London: RCS.

Shah S (1999) Neurological assessment. Nursing Standard 13(22): 49–54.

Teasdale G, Jennett B (1974) Assessment of coma and impaired consciousness. A practical scale. Lancet ii: 81–4.

United Kingdom Central Council for Nursing, Midwifery and Health Visiting (1992) Code of Professional Conduct for the Nurse, Midwife and Health Visitor. London: UKCC.

CHAPTER 7

Special cases and complications

TOM CRIPPS

Although gastroenterological endoscopy is usually considered to be a safe procedure, numerous adverse events have been described in association with both the procedure itself and the sedative techniques used to facilitate it. Many of the complications of sedation for endoscopy (for example, hypoxaemia) can also occur in the absence of sedation. As the author takes the viewpoint that sedationists will be responsible for the overall physiological welfare of their patients, this chapter will discuss any problems that the sedationist is likely to encounter and should be able to manage even if these are not necessarily caused by the sedation itself.

The chapter is laid out as follows:

1. Classification and incidence of complications;
2. Complications associated with the technique of intravenous injection;
3. Side effects and complications of sedative drugs;
4. Cardiorespiratory complications;
5. Other medical problems during endoscopy;
6. Important surgical complications of endoscopy;
7. Risk management: how sedationists can optimize patient safety;
8. Summary and conclusion.

Figures 7.1–7.10 complement the text and are designed to provide the sedationists with a framework on which to build their own protocols for preventing and dealing with complications, adapted to the particular skill mix and patient population of their individual endoscopy unit.

Classification and incidence of complications

The real incidence of complications is difficult to establish because the published data tend to be retrospective (and therefore subject to underreporting), vary in terms of what is defined as a complication, and refer to large individual studies by particularly enthusiastic and highly experienced operators. Cotton and Williams (1996) make the point that some adverse events would be better classified as 'incidents' since they are of no long-term consequence if properly managed. Complications can be classified according to the body system that is affected (for example, cardiovascular or respiratory), the cause of the problem or its implications for the patient or for completion of the procedure.

Fleischer et al. (1997) have devised a new system for the classification of complications that grades the immediate negative outcome (O), long-term disability (D) and death (D). This ODD system separates events that have potentially harmful consequences if not properly managed (for example, hypoxaemia) from actual harmful outcomes, and quantifies the importance of these outcomes. Such a system can be tailored to the individual endoscopy unit as a basis of audit and risk management.

Most reported series quote an incidence of serious morbidity of approximately 1 per 1000 for endoscopies, with a mortality of perhaps 1 in 2000, and claim that most of these are caused by cardiorespiratory complications (British Society of Gastroenterology, 1991; Benjamin, 1996; Chan, 1996; Cotton and Williams, 1996), but the frequency of incidents that could potentially lead to a life-threatening complication if not properly managed is far higher.

Complications associated with the technique of intravenous injection

Problems with intravenous access include:

1. failed cannulation;
2. haematoma;
3. infection;
4. phlebitis;
5. painful injection;
6. intra-arterial injection;
7. air embolism;
8. the cannula not having been removed.

Most of these complications are preventable, should be rare and of little long-term consequence and should be avoidable by using a good technique and sound departmental protocols (see Chapters 4 and 8).

Because it is water soluble, midazolam is not usually associated with phlebitis. Similarly, intra-arterial injection with midazolam (albeit undesirable) is usually devoid of long-term sequelae; any suspicion of this should, however, prompt an immediate cessation of injection, a change of venepuncture site and careful observation.

Side effects and complications of sedative drugs

Any drug can produce unwanted effects by a number of different mechanisms. Type A reactions are an extension of the normal pharmacological response, relatively common and dose related (Association of Anaesthetists and British Society of Allergy and Clinical Immunology, 1995):

1. *An exaggerated pharmacological response*: an actual or relative overdose of the drug results in a greater than expected response, as seen with general anaesthesia induced by midazolam injection.
2. *An unusual or paradoxical response*: the patient responds in an unusual way, but this response is recognized to occur in some patients and is explained by the drug's mechanism of action. Examples here are drug interactions, the patient displaying agitation rather than sedation, and the erotic fantasies associated with midazolam use (Dundee et al., 1991).

Type B reactions are not dose related and can be precipitated by a tiny quantity of a drug. They tend to become worse on repeated exposure and are not typical 'pharmacological' responses. This is typical of an immunological cause. These can be *allergic reactions*, for example anaphylaxis.

Of all these reactions, the type A dose-related effects, directly predictable from a knowledge of the pharmacological effects of midazolam, are by far the most common. These include:

1. respiratory depression leading to hypoxaemia, hypercarbia and ultimately respiratory arrest;
2. cardiovascular depression and vasodilatation leading to hypotension;
3. a loss of protective reflexes, leading to pulmonary aspiration.

Because the brainstem, and thus the control of breathing and circulation, is 'sedated', it is quite predictable that midazolam and other sedative drugs will cause some respiratory and cardiovascular depression. This is exacerbated by the use of other depressants (for example opioids) or by abolishing the protective reflexes with local anaesthesia. Sedationists must be aware of these potential complications, first ensuring that their technique prevents these wherever possible, and second recognizing them should they occur despite this. The treatment of these problems is outlined below and illustrated in Figures 7.1–7.7.

The interaction between the sedative drug and the patient may also give unexpected results: in some cases, midazolam appears to have little or no effect even in generous doses. This is particularly likely in patients whose receptors are desensitized because they are regularly taking large doses of benzodiazepines for other reasons, and in drug and alcohol addicts; sedation may require the use of another category of drug, for example propofol. Other patients do not respond to conscious sedation by co-operating with the procedure. There are two probable causes for this: patients may be unable to co-operate for physical or psychological reasons (and are therefore unsuitable for conscious sedation), or they may have become oversedated. In either situation, it is pointless and dangerous to continue to administer a sedative (see Chapter 4).

Immunological reactions to drugs can be localized or systemic. A localized reaction is usually manifested by itching, erythema (redness) or swelling at the site of injection and along the vein. A localized reaction rarely needs to be treated. In contrast, an anaphylactic reaction is life-threatening. Anaphylaxis is the result of the body's immune system recognizing a foreign substance and mounting a massive response against it. This response involves the release of histamine and other vasoactive amines into the circulation and, rather than protecting patients, can actually kill them. The features of an anaphylactic reaction and its treatment are summarised in Figure 7.1.

It should be noted that an anaphylactic reaction can be caused by any foreign substance that patients receive in association with endoscopy, and prior uneventful exposure, far from indicating that patients will not demonstrate an allergic reaction, actually gives them the chance to become sensitized. Although such a reaction can be caused by a sedative or analgesic drug, it can equally easily be caused by local anaesthetic spray, a prophylactic antibiotic or – increasingly – latex gloves.

Although anaphylactic reactions are uncommon during endoscopy, the sedationist must be able to recognize them and initiate prompt treatment

---

Possible causes during endoscopy
- Sedative drugs, opioids
- Local anaesthetics
- Antibiotics
- Latex

Incidence during endoscopy
- Unknown, possibly 1 in 10 000

Consequences
- Respiratory and circulatory failure
- May be rapidly fatal if not properly treated

Prevention
- Careful medical history – avoid known allergens

Diagnosis
Affects one or more of the body systems. The sooner a reaction is observed after exposure to a foreign substance, the more severe it tends to be. The percentages below refer to the approximate proportion of patients having an anaphylactic reaction who will display those signs (Association of Anaesthetists and British Society of Allergy and Clinical Immunology, 1995).
- *Cardiovascular system* (88%): hypotension, tachycardia, circulatory collapse, death. NB: Tachycardia and hypotension are a feature of anaphylaxis; vasovagal responses are associated with bradycardia
- *Respiratory system* (36%): bronchospasm, breathlessness, stridor, hypoxaemia
- *Angio-oedema* (24%): swelling of the face, tongue and upper airway
- *Skin* (50%): erythema, swelling, rash, itch
- *Gastrointestinal system:* nausea, vomiting, abdominal cramps (diarrhoea)
- *Central nervous system:* anxiety, confusion, unconsciousness

Figure 7.1 Anaphylaxis.

for what is, in these circumstances, a totally iatrogenic condition. Any delay in the administration of adrenaline (epinephrine) reduces the chance of recovery. The optimal dosage regimen is debatable, but departmental protocols should follow the advice given in the current edition of the *British National Formulary* or that of similarly authoritative sources such as the UK Resuscitation Council (2002) and the Association of Anaesthetists (Association of Anaesthetists and British Society of Allergy and Clinical Immunology, 1995).

Cardiorespiratory complications

As stated above, cardiopulmonary problems can occur during endoscopy even in the absence of sedation. Indeed, sedation may protect a patient from some complications by reducing anxiety and the associated cardiovascular responses related to it. Eckhardt et al. (1999), for example, studying patients undergoing colonoscopy who were selected either to receive or not receive sedation, observed about twice the incidence of oxygen desaturation when sedation was used, but vasovagal reactions, some of which were considered life-threatening, were more frequent in the absence of sedation; none of the episodes of desaturation was considered life-threatening.

Respiratory problems include:

1. hypoxaemia;
2. respiratory depression;
3. respiratory arrest;
4. pulmonary aspiration of gastric contents.

Hypoxaemia describes a fall in the oxygen concentration (or saturation) of the arterial blood. It should be noted that the oxygen saturation must fall to below 85–90% for cyanosis (blueness) to be detected by eye; decreases of a lesser degree cannot be detected without using a pulse oximeter. Studies during endoscopy frequently define hypoxaemia as a fall in oxygen saturation to below 90% or a fall of greater than 4% below baseline. Using this definition, hypoxaemia is extremely common, occurring in as many as half of all patients breathing room air while undergoing endoscopy. The causes for this are not fully understood as although it is observed more frequently when a patient is sedated, is undergoing upper endoscopy or has intercurrent disease, it still occurs in the absence of these factors.

It is unlikely that transient hypoxaemia of this degree, albeit undesirable, is in itself harmful to a patient, but a lowered saturation does, however, indicate that there is respiratory compromise. Hypoxaemia is of course a frequent manifestation of respiratory depression. It is, however, possible for serious ventilatory inadequacy to be present in the absence of arterial desaturation if a patient is receiving supplemental oxygen; this is most probable in the small group of patients with chronic airways disease who have become dependent on hypoxaemia for their respiratory drive. The sedationist must therefore always be alert to other respiratory parameters (rate, depth and pattern) in addition to oxygen saturation and cyanosis. By close attention to the patient's clinical state, it is possible to anticipate and correct the vast majority of problems associated with hypoxaemia and respiratory depression before they progress to a respiratory arrest or other life-threatening emergency. An approach to the prevention, diagnosis and treatment of these problems is outlined in Figure 7.2.

Possible causes during endoscopy
· Sedative drugs (benzodiazepines, opioids)
· Mechanical and reflex effects of the endoscope
· Secondary to cardiovascular problems
· Existing medical/respiratory conditions
· Rare mechanical problems (e.g. pneumothorax)
· Anaphylaxis, aspiration

Incidence during endoscopy
· Hypoxaemia in >50% of sedated patients breathing air; also observed in the absence of sedation
· Supplemental oxygen reduces hypoxaemic episodes but not respiratory depression

Consequences
· May progress to respiratory arrest
· Hypoxaemia can cause myocardial ischaemia
· Respiratory depression increases risk of pulmonary aspiration

Prevention
· Avoid oversedation
· Special care for patients with pre-existing disease
· Meticulous monitoring of respiratory status
· Supplemental oxygen reduces hypoxaemic episodes but not respiratory depression

Diagnosis
· Fall in oxygen saturation (requires pulse oximetry)
· Cyanosis (unlikely to detect hypoxaemia until SpO_2 is < 85-90%
· Reduced respiratory rate or depth
· Unconscious / unresponsive

Actions
· Conscious patient
   - Encourage deep breathing
   - Consider supplemental oxygen
   - Reduce sedation
· Unconscious patient
   - Inform operator
   - Discontinue procedure
   - Check Airway, Breathing, Circulation (CPR IF APPROPRIATE)
   - Oxygen, assist respiration
   - Reverse sedation : antagonists – Flumazenil, Naloxone

Figure 7.2 Hypoxaemia and respiratory depression.

The pulmonary aspiration of gastric contents is relatively common after upper gastrointestinal endoscopy (Chan, 1996). However, whereas it has been demonstrated experimentally in more than a third of patients undergoing routine endoscopy, the incidence of clinically significant aspiration is far less – of the order of 1 in 1000. Aspiration can lead to immediate respiratory distress and asphyxia, aspiration pneumonitis, adult respiratory distress syndrome and aspiration pneumonia. Anything that depresses the respiratory reflexes or increases the volume of the stomach contents increases the risk of aspiration. Risk factors therefore include active upper gastrointestinal bleeding or bowel obstruction, and patients whose reflexes are depressed by pharyngeal anaesthesia, sedative drugs or their medical condition (for example, stroke or liver failure.) There is a strong correlation between the use of local anaesthetic sprays and the subsequent development of pneumonia (Quine et al., 1995). It is strongly advisable to recruit an anaesthetist to protect the airway in those at highest risk. An approach to preventing and treating pulmonary aspiration is shown in Figure 7.3.

Cardiovascular problems include:

1. hypotension;
2. vasovagal events;
3. myocardial ischaemia;
4. cardiac arrhythmia;
5. cardiac arrest.

There are four separate influences on a patient's cardiovascular system during endoscopy:

1. the patient's underlying medical condition: the presence or absence of heart disease, hypertension and so on, and the relevant medications;
2. any acute physiological changes such as gastrointestinal haemorrhage;
3. surgical stimulation from the endoscopic procedure;
4. the effect of sedative and other drugs administered during the procedure.

The sedationist must interpret any cardiovascular events occurring during endoscopy with these factors in mind if they are to be managed correctly.

Hypotension refers to a fall in blood pressure and should be defined with respect to the patient's normal pressure – for example, as a fall of greater than 30% – rather than by setting an arbitrary level such as 100 mmHg

Possible causes during endoscopy
- Full stomach
  - Inadequate starvation
  - Active bleeding
  - Bowel obstruction
- Depressed reflexes
  - Sedation; pharyngeal local anaesthetic
  - Neurological problems (stroke, myopathy, etc.)
  - Reduced consciousness
  - General debility
- Positioning during and after procedure

Incidence during endoscopy
- Aspiration can be demonstrated in up to 33% of patients undergoing upper gastrointestinal endoscopy
- 1 in 1000 cases develop serious consequences

Consequences
- Acute respiratory distress
- Aspiration pneumonia
- Aspiration pneumonitis – adult respiratory distress syndrome
- Asphyxia (overwhelming volume)

Prevention
- Avoid oversedation; caution with local anaesthetic spray
- Identify high-risk patients
- Avoid full stomach if possible
- Safe positioning, generous pharyngeal suction
- Use endotracheal tube in high-risk patients

Diagnosis
- Direct observation of event
- Hypoxaemia and respiratory distress, bronchospasm
- Presentation may be immediate or delayed (pneumonia)

Actions
- Immediate:
  - Check airway, breathing, circulation
  - Put in safe position, suction
  - Oxygen
  - Stop/reverse sedative and opioid drugs
- Observe
- Consult physician / intensivist

Figure 7.3 Pulmonary aspiration.

systolic, since a blood pressure that is normal for one patient may be dangerously low for one who is usually hypertensive. The significance of a fall in blood pressure depends on the whole clinical picture. It is in most instances benign, merely reflecting a well-sedated patient, but it is important to discriminate conditions requiring intervention, such as vasovagal reactions, rhythm disturbances, hypovolaemia and anaphylaxis. An approach to the diagnosing and treatment of hypotension is shown in Figure 7.4.

Vasovagal reactions are caused by activation of the vagus nerve in response to physical or emotional events. Fainting is the typical vasovagal response observed in a conscious, upright patient and is characterized by pallor, sweating, bradycardia, hypotension and ultimately loss of consciousness as a result of an insufficient cerebral blood supply. Autonomic reflexes, and pain caused by visceral distension, are the most probable causes of a vasovagal response during endoscopy. Although there is some evidence that sedation actually reduces the risk of such a reaction, vasovagal responses may be observed in over 10% of patients undergoing colonoscopy with sedation (M.Henderson, personal communication, 2001). Vasovagal responses are usually self-limiting provided that they are recognized and the initiating stimulus is removed, although active treatment is occasionally required. The diagnosis and management of vasovagal responses is summarised in Figure 7.5.

Cardiac arrhythmias and myocardial ischaemia are relatively common during endoscopy, some studies reporting arrhythmias in over half of the subjects and myocardial ischaemia in over one-third; these disturbances tend to be more common in patients with pre-existing cardiopulmonary disease. In these studies, 'arrhythmias' may include sinus tachycardia and ventricular and supraventricular extrasystoles, which are frequently considered to be benign, and 'myocardial ischaemia' is defined by depression of the ST segments on the ECG. Most of these episodes are asymptomatic with no long-term sequelae, but a minority are associated with anginal chest pain or haemodynamically significant arrhythmias. Myocardial infarction, heart failure and cardiac arrest are rare but have occasionally been reported.

It is often claimed that the cause of myocardial ischaemia during endoscopy is hypoxaemia, but since only a minority of cases of myocardial ischaemia are associated with simultaneous hypoxaemia, this is, at the very least, a gross oversimplification. Myocardial ischaemia reflects an imbalance between myocardial oxygen demand and supply. Hypoxaemia reduces oxygen supply, as does hypotension (although the latter also

Possible causes during endoscopy
- Sedation – cardiovascular depression and vasodilatation
- Vasovagal
- Hypovolaemia (bleeding)
- Anaphylaxis
- Myocardial ischaemia / heart failure
- Septicaemia – pre-existing or caused by procedure

Incidence during endoscopy
- Up to 10% of cases, depending on definition and underlying condition
- <1% require major interventions

Consequences
- Usually benign but may cause major complications in patients with cardiovascular disease
- Delay in discharge from the unit
- Myocardial ischaemia, cardiac arrhythmias, coronary thrombosis
- Cerebral ischaemia, stroke
- Renal failure

Prevention
- Avoid oversedation
- Emergency cases properly resuscitated
- Special care in high risk cases :
  - Ischaemic heart disease / cerebrovascular disease
  - Emergency cases
  - Surgical cases with a risk of bleeding (e.g. sphincterotomy, varices)

Diagnosis
- Blood pressure recording. Diagnosis requires a *percentage fall* below patient's normal (preprocedure) blood pressure
- Clinical Monitoring - weak pulse, poor oximetry trace
- Agitation, confusion

Actions
- Check Airway, Breathing, Circulation
- Establish **cause** and **significance** and **treat appropriately** for example:
  - No treatment
  - Discontinue endoscopy, deflate stomach or bowel
  - Stop, reduce or reverse sedation
  - Intravenous fluids for hypovolaemia or blood loss
  - Vasovagal reaction (Figure 7.5)
  - Anaphylaxis (Figure 7.1)
  - Myocardial Ischaemia – Nitrates

Figure 7.4 Hypotension.

Possible causes during endoscopy
- Anxiety
- Pain
- Autonomic – overinflated viscus and stretching mesentery

Incidence during endoscopy
- Observed in up to 10% of colonoscopies (rarer in upper gastrointestinal endoscopy)
- 1 in 100 cases require significant intervention
- Up to 20% of colonoscopic complications

Consequences
- Usually resolves without sequelae if treated properly
- Myocardial and Cerebral Ischaemia
- Procedure may need to be abandoned

Prevention
- Gentle, skilful endoscopy
- Avoid overdistension of viscus or traction on mesentery
- Reassurance and sedation
- Atropine or similar anticholinergic drug

Diagnosis
- Bradycardia
- Hypotension
- Pallor and sweating
- Loss of consciousness (fainting) if head is raised
- Differentiate from other causes of hypotension (Figure 7.4)

Actions
- Check Airway, Breathing, Circulation
- Raise legs, lie flat
- Reverse causative stimuli:
    - Deflate viscus
    - Stop bowel traction
    - Discontinue endoscopy
- If condition does not improve rapidly, consider:
    - administration of atropine
    - fluid therapy

Figure 7.5 Vasovagal reaction.

reduces oxygen demand). Anything, however, that increases oxygen demand, such as hypertension caused by surgical stimulation or anxiety, and tachycardia resulting from these same factors as well as the administration of anticholinergic drugs such as hyoscine butylbromide (Buscopan), may be more important, particularly when acting at the same time as hypoxaemia. There is also evidence that upper gastrointesntinal

Possible causes during endoscopy
- Pre-existing heart disease
- Anxiety, pain
- Secondary to respiratory depression (hypoxaemia, hypercarbia)
- Hypotension, hypertension and tachycardia, especially in patients with ischaemic heart disease

Incidence during endoscopy
- Reported in up to 50% of cases depending on case mix
- Life-threatening disturbances are relatively rare

Consequences
- Ischaemia can lead to life-threatening arrhythmias and myocardial infarction
- Arrhythmias can lead to haemodynamic compromise, myocardial ischaemia and cardiac arrest

Prevention
- Careful assessment and preparation of high-risk patients:
  - Ischaemic heart disease
  - Recent infarction
  - Severe valvular disease
- Prevent hypoxaemia (Figure 7.2)
- Avoid tachycardia in high-risk patients (consider beta blockers)

Diagnosis
- Ischaemia
  - S-T segment changes on ECG
  - Anginal Chest Pain
- Arrhythmia:
  - Irregular pulse, bradycardia or tachycardia
  - Rhythm changes on ECG

Actions
- Check Airway, Breathing, Circulation
- Treat hypoxaemia – administer oxygen
- Treat causes of hypotension (if possible)
- Alert operator and stop procedure
- Refer to physician if condition persists

Figure 7.6 Myocardial ischaemia, cardiac arrhythmia.

endoscopy can in itself cause myocardial ischaemia through viscerocardiac reflexes (Holm and Rosenberg, 1996). An approach to diagnosing and treating myocardial ischaemia and rhythm disturbances is shown in Figure 7.6.

Cardiac arrests are very uncommon during endoscopy but can occur as a result of any of the influences described at the beginning of this section.

The sedationist should aim to manage the patient's condition in order to avoid cardiorespiratory events progressing to a cardiac arrest, and should anticipate an increased risk in those who suffer from severe pre-existing heart disease or recent myocardial infarction. The standard of care should anticipate and wherever possible prevent a cardiac arrest. It is essential that the whole team has a well-practised and effective plan for dealing with one, should it occur, and that each member receives regular resuscitation updates. In the UK and Europe, resuscitation is practised in a standardized manner according to the guidelines of the UK and European Resuscitation Councils (European Resuscitation Council, 1998a, 1998b; Resuscitation Council UK, 2000), similar guidelines existing in other countries. Although it is not intended to reproduce these here, it is important to discuss the *level* of resuscitation expertise available to the endoscopy team:

1. As in any healthcare setting, all staff must be proficient in basic life support.
2. Members of the endoscopy team must be able to oxygenate the patient with the aid of a bag-valve-mask and oropharyngeal airway ± laryngeal mask airway.
3. A member of the team must be trained, able and willing to defibrillate a patient who has a shockable cardiac arrest rhythm (that is, ventricular fibrillation or pulseless ventricular tachycardia).
4. There must be immediate access to advanced life support, either a member of the endoscopy team who is trained in this or the cardiac arrest team.

The level of training required by sedationists depends on the skill mix of the whole endoscopy team, but as a minimum they should have attained level 2, and preferably level 3, in the list above. Figure 7.7 summarises an approach to the prevention, recognition and management of cardiac arrest.

Other medical problems during endoscopy

Patients frequently suffer from intercurrent disease, endoscopy often being performed because of gastroenterological problems associated with or presenting during their care for another condition. These conditions may require management or lead to complications during endscopy. Examples of these conditions and their management are shown in Figure 7.8.

Skill levels - description
1. Basic life support (Resuscitation Council[a])
   - Basic recognition and treatment of cardiac and respiratory arrest
   - Airway Breathing Circulation
2. Intermediate level 1
   - Bag – mask – airway ventilation (± laryngeal mask airway)
   - Oxygen administration
3. Intermediate level 2
   - Defibrillation
4. Advanced life support (Resuscitation Council[a])

Suggested skills for endoscopy team[b]
1. Basic life support
   - All members of endoscopy team
2. Bag – mask – airway ventilation; oxygen administration
   - All members of team (± laryngeal mask airway)
3. Defibrillation
   - Skilled practitioner always in team, preferably sedationist
4. Advanced life support
   - Immediately available (cardiac arrest team)
   - Ideally skill within endoscopy team

Training
Life support training in a simulated emergency working as a team
   - Minimum annual updates of theoretical training; preferably 6-monthly
   - Regularly test ability to summon arrest team and response times

a   UK / European Resuscitation Guidelines for Basic and Advanced Life Support are recommended (see text)
b   Life support skills required will depend on the exact skill mix of the endoscopy team as well as organization
    of the unit and proximity to Hospital cardiac arrest team.

Figure 7.7 Resuscitation skills for the endoscopy team.

Important surgical complications of endoscopy

Because endoscopy is an invasive procedure, there are inevitably problems and complications associated with the procedure itself, such as bowel perforation, sepsis and haemorrhage. If therapeutic procedures are also performed, the incidence of these complications is much increased. The protocols drawn up for the whole endoscopy process need to reflect these possible complications and ensure that they are detected and managed as appropriately as possible. The complications are sometimes first recognized by the sedationist; some of these are listed in Figure 7.9.

Risk management: how sedationists can optimize patient safety

It should be clear that although there are many potentially serious complications of sedation and endoscopy, events such as moderate

Indications for endoscopy which increase the risks of sedation:
- Acute gastrointestinal bleeding (shock; aspiration)
- Liver failure, varices (altered consciousness; bleeding)
- Thrombolysis (following myocardial infarction: high cardiac risk)
- Bowel obstruction (aspiration)
- Stroke, head injury, brain damage (percutaneous endoscopic gastrotomy: altered consciousness – respiratory depression and aspiration risk)

Examples of intercurrent medical problems that increase risks from sedation and endoscopy
- Respiratory disease:
  - Asthma, chronic obstructive airways disease (may be exacerbated during procedure; sedation more likely to cause respiratory depression; limited reserve)
- Cardiovascular disease
  - Ischaemic heart disease, recent myocardial infarction (increased risk of ischaemia and rhythm disturbance)
  - Valvular and congenital heart disease (haemodynamic effects of the procedure and sedation can be serious)
  - Heart failure, cardiomyopathy
- Endocrine
  - Diabetes requiring insulin (risk of hypoglycaemia and unconsciousness – needs good blood glucose management)
  - Adrenal suppression (steroids) or deficiency (risk of hypotension if not adequately managed)
- Neurological disease
  - Stroke, obtunded consciousness, myopathy (increased risk of aspiration and respiratory failure)
  - Epilepsy (risk of seizure)
- Haematological disease
  - Anaemia (less tolerant of hypoxaemia)
  - Coagulopathy / thrombocytopenia (bleeding risk)
- Liver disease
  - Drug metabolism altered, encephalopathy, coagulopathy
- Renal disease
  - Drug metabolism altered, cardiovascular problems
- Drug therapy
  - May alter response to sedative drugs
- Frail / elderly

Figure 7.8 Existing medical problems and sedation for endoscopy.

hypoxaemia or myocardial ischaemia indeed being common, the actual incidence of serious harm is low. Sedationists must ensure that their practices will whenever possible anticipate and prevent complications, and allow prompt and effective treatment if they do occur. A strategy to achieve this has two aspects.

- **Pain and discomfort**
  - Vasovagal reactions
  - Encourages oversedation
  - Reflects surgical complication (e.g. perforation)
- **Bleeding**
  - Hypotension, myocardial ischaemia, shock
- **Infection**
  - Septicaemia – hypotension and collapse
- **Pneumothorax, pneumoperitoneum**
  - Respiratory distress, hypoxaemia, cardiovascular compromise
- **Venous air embolism**
  - Circulatory collapse

Figure 7.9 Surgical complications of endoscopy and their relevance to the sedationist.

First, ensure that the sedation technique is safe and meticulous. In particular, do not oversedate the patient. If the procedure cannot be completed with conscious sedation, it should be abandoned. A general anaesthetic should be requested from a *trained anaesthetist*, and the sedationist needs to be assertive enough to say 'no' however demanding the operator is.

Second, it is possible to identify those patients who are at highest risk of complications in order to ensure that they are treated with extra precautions. Figure 7.10 lists categories of patient who carry the highest risk. The American Society of Anesthesiologists (1963) assessment has also been found to identify groups of patient at increased risk of complications during endoscopy (Alcain et al., 1998; Eckhardt et al., 1999) and has been proposed by the British Society of Gastroenterology (1991). The Hvidovre endoscopy risk score is a similar system proposed by Holm and Rosenberg (1996). Once high-risk patients have been identified, the endoscopy team has to decide how they can best be managed. This will vary according to the available skill mix but might involve the use of extra monitoring, supplemental oxygen, the avoidance of sedation and the recruitment of an anaesthetist (Figure 7.10).

Summary and conclusion

1. Serious morbidity and death in association with endoscopy are rare occurences but events that can potentially lead to serious complications if they are not properly managed are common.
2. Complications associated with endoscopy are underreported, and their actual incidence is unknown.

Categories of high-risk patient
- Severe respiratory disease, respiratory failure
- Depressed consciousness
- Depressed respiratory reflexes
- Severe heart disease
  - Ischaemic (unstable angina, recent myocardial infarction)
  - Cardiomyopathy
  - Valvular / congenital
  - Heart failure
- Active bleeding in upper gastrointestinal tract
- Full stomach for other reason
- Haemodynamically unstable / shocked
- Emergency cases with other underlying pathologies
- Known difficulty with procedure or sedation
- Frail elderly
- ASA III / IV patients (see text)

Management strategies
- Consider appropriateness of procedure
- Delay until condition has been optimized
- Consider avoiding all sedation
  - Do not be bullied into giving sedation when it is unsafe
  - Do not be bullied into oversedating a patient
- Increase level of monitoring and support
  - Additional oxygen
  - Continuous oximetry, ECG, blood pressure
- Use anaesthetist and full operating theatre facilities

Figure 7.10 Identification of patients at high risk of complication during sedation and endoscopy.

3. The sedationist must be able to recognize and treat all life-threatening emergencies that occur during endoscopy and not just those caused by sedation.
4. It is possible to identify patients most at risk of complications and take appropriate precautions.
5. Cardiopulmonary problems contribute a high proportion of the serious complications associated with endoscopy. These problems can be minimized but not totally eliminated by careful monitoring and the avoidance of oversedation.
6. The endoscopy team must have appropriate resuscitation skills and practise these regularly in simulated emergencies.

Acknowledgement

The author acknowledges the invaluable help and advice provided by Morag Henderson, Endoscopy Sister at the Borders General Hospital, during preparation of this chapter. Thanks also to Mr Colin Murray, Resuscitation Training Officer and Staff Nurse Ronnie Dornan for their comments on the manuscript.

References

Alcain G, Guillen P, Moreno M, Martin L (1998) Predictive factors of oxygen desaturation during upper gastrointestinal endoscopy in nonsedated patients. Gastrointestinal Endoscopy 48(2): 143–7.

American Society of Anesthesiologists (1963) New classification of physical status. Anesthesiology 24: 111.

Association of Anaesthetists of Great Britain and Ireland and British Society of Allergy and Clinical Immunology (1995) Suspected Anaphylactic Reactions Associated with Anaesthesia. London: AAGBI.

Benjamin SB (1996) Complications of conscious sedation. Gastrointestinal Endoscopy Clinics of North America 6(2): 277–85.

British National Formulary. London: BMJ Books, regularly updated.

British Society of Gastroenterology (1991) British Society of Gastroenterology recommendations for standards of sedation and patient monitoring during gastrointestinal endoscopy. Gut 32: 823–7.

Chan MF (1996) Complications of upper gastrointestinal endoscopy. Gastrointestinal Endoscopy Clinics of North America 6(2): 287–303.

Cotton P, Williams C (1996) Practical Gastrointestinal Endoscopy. Oxford: Blackwell Science.

Dundee JW, Clarke RSJ, McCaughey (1991) Clinical Anaesthetic Pharmacology. Edinburgh: Churchill Livingstone.

Eckhardt VF, Kanzler G, Schmitt T, Eckhardt J, Bernhard G (1999) Complications and adverse effects of colonoscopy with selective sedation. Gastrointestinal Endoscopy 49(5): 560–5.

European Resuscitation Council (1998a) European Resuscitation Council guidelines for adult advanced life support. Resuscitation 37: 81–90.

European Resuscitation Council (1998b) European Resuscitation Council guidelines for adult single rescuer basic life support. Resuscitation 37: 67–80.

Fleischer DE, Mierop FV, Eisen GM et al. (1997) A new system for defining endoscopic complications emphasising the measure of importance. Gastrointestinal Endoscopy 45(2): 128–33.

Holm C, Rosenberg J (1996) Pulse oximetry and supplemental oxygen during gastrointestinal endoscopy: a critical review. Endoscopy 28: 703–11.

Quine MA, Bell GD, McCloy RF, Charlton JE, Devlin HB, Hopkins A (1995) Prospective audit of upper gastrointestinal endoscopy in two regions of England: safety, staffing and sedation methods. Gut 36(3): 462–7.

Resuscitation Council UK (2000) Resuscitation Guidelines 2000. London: Resuscitation Council [The most recent resuscitation protocols can be accessed at the Resuscitation Council website www.resus.org.uk].

Resuscitation Council UK (2002) Emergency Medical Treatment of Anaphylactic Reactions for First Medical Responders and Community Nurses. Revised January 2002. London: Resuscitation Council [The most recent resuscitation protocols can be accessed at the Resuscitation Council website www.resus.org.uk].

CHAPTER 8

Professional and legal aspects

DIANE PALMER

The aim of this chapter is to consider professional and legal issues directly related to the administration of intravenous conscious sedation. Relevant aspects of the nurses' *Code of Professional Conduct* (NMC, 2002a) will be identified and issues of accountability and liability in relation to the expanded role explored. The administration of medicines under the direction of group protocols, nurse prescribing and the United Kingdom Central Council for Nursing, Midwifery and Health Visiting (UKCC) recommendations for the 'higher-level practitioner' will be discussed. Readers should, however, be aware that developments in legislation occur almost continually, and it is therefore necessary for individuals to monitor guidelines and recommendations produced by bodies such as the Department of Health (DoH), the Nursing and Midwifery Council (NMC) and the Royal Colleges.

Code of Professional Conduct

The UKCC document *Scope of Professional Practice* (1992) was an initiative to facilitate the expansion of the role of the nurse. One of the main recommendations arising from this document was that the focus for developments should be professional accountability and responsibility rather than the previous certificate of competence for a task. Nurses now carry out many procedures previously undertaken by medical staff, but there are concerns that nurses may be required to undertake tasks beyond their professional competence or work beyond the confines of algorithm guidelines and group protocols. This probably results from a failure to understand the limitations of the nurses' Code of Conduct (NMC, 2002a) and possibly from the constraints of severe staff shortage leading to stressful working conditions and inappropriate demands.

Every professional group is accountable to a governing body. The NMC governs nurses in the UK, providing standards and guidelines for professional practice and conduct (NMC, 2002a). Nurses undertaking expanded and advanced practice roles should have received appropriate education and training to support this development, ideally at an approved higher educational institution or education centre. All nurses and midwives are expected regularly to take part in learning activities, which develop competence and performance while acknowledging aspects of practice beyond the practitioners' levels and competence, and obtaining help and supervision when necessary (NMC, 2002a).

Accountability and liability

The nurse is legally, ethically, morally and professionally bound, which can, when considered and analysed, be daunting. A breach of legal duty of care will deem a nurse negligent, but negligence claims need to determine that the nurse has practised to a standard not accepted as proper by a responsible body of nursing opinion (*Bolam* v. *Friern Hospital Management Committee* 1957). So the nurse who maintains an adequate standard of care and makes decisions based on professional judgement from a sound knowledge base should have little to fear. Accidents do happen, and there are obviously events and circumstances that cannot be predicted or controlled. Clinical practice incorporating a risk assessment and reduction approach will, however, identify when predicted risk may occur and should do much to reduce the threat of negligence.

The boundary between responsibility and appropriateness of delegation has generated some confusion. Whereas some medical staff are unclear about when care can be allocated to a non-medical practitioner, non-medical staff have concerns that they may be extending their professional boundaries beyond their level of practice. The General Medical Council (GMC) guidelines, however, clearly state that care can be delegated to healthcare staff who are not medical practitioners if it is in the best interests of the patient (GMC, 1995). The medical practitioner remains responsible for the management of the patient's care and must not delegate a task which requires the knowledge and skills of a doctor (GMC, 1995), while always ensuring that the person to whom the procedure is delegated is sufficiently competent.

Common sense would advise that managers and doctors should not force nurses to expand their role beyond their capabilities: this could result in poor standards of practice, stress or illness. If, however, the professional standard for a particular post requires an expanded role, the post-holder will be expected to perform and operate with the skill and competence equivalent to that of other such post-holders. If a nurse takes on a role previously carried out by a doctor, he or she will be judged by the same standard as the doctor. Competence to perform the role should thus be at a level equivalent to that of a medical practitioner. If a nurse were accused of negligence, the excuse of inexperience would not be accepted as a defence by either the General Medical Council or the UK legal system. The law requires students and novices to be judged by the same standards as experienced practitioners, and it is a requirement of the NMC (2002a) that the nurse take steps to rectify any knowledge deficits by regularly taking part in learning activities.

It is acceptable for non-medical practitioners to expand their practice to include the administration of intravenous sedation if they have received appropriate and adequate education and training, but the sedation must be administered within the boundaries of the practitioner's knowledge and training. Patients assessed utilizing the American Society of Anesthesiologists (ASA) criteria who are classified as group I or II are unlikely to require the knowledge of a doctor while receiving their sedation and can be adequately cared for by a practitioner who has received appropriate education and achieved a level of competency in practice. Patients in ASA classes III–V are, however, likely to require intensive management while receiving sedation and are therefore not an appropriate group to be cared for solely by a non-medical practitioner.

When a doctor delegates a task, he or she may still, according to the 'captain of the ship' approach, be ultimately responsible (Montgomery, 1992), but it is the nurse's responsibility to ensure that guidelines for practice are agreed with the medical practitioner and carried out accordingly. Any breach of the practice guidelines will obviously be deemed potentially negligent, and the doctor cannot be held responsible. If practice guidelines are breached in adverse circumstances when professional judgement has had to be applied and initiated, the practitioner will have to justify his or her actions. If a negligence claim were to be made following actions lying outside the agreed guidelines, the nurse would have to prove that, in similar circumstances, a medical practitioner would have acted in a similar manner.

Standards for the administration of medicines

It is the nurses' responsibility to ensure that, when they are involved in the administration of medicines, appropriate knowledge, skill and judgement are applied. The nurse must have a clear understanding of the medicines used and be able to judge the suitability of the prescription for the patient at that time (NMC, 2002b).

Nurse prescribing

The subject of nurse prescribing appears to have been on the 'developments in nursing' agenda for many years. It was back in 1986 that Baroness Julia Cumberlege first suggested that community nurses should have prescribing rights, particularly for appliances and dressings. At the time of publication, several sites are evaluating nurses' prescribing from a formulary, as described by the Crown Report (DoH, 1999a).

The current legislation does not permit nurses to prescribe any medications not listed in the nurse prescriber's formulary. Practice has, however, evolved such that many nurses with the appropriate education and competence are administering medications in accordance with drug protocols that have been developed under the guidance of medical practitioners.

Patient group directions

Many nurses now administer medications as directed from drug protocols that are now referred to in legal terms as 'patient group directions' (PGDs) (National Assembly for Wales, 2000; National Health Service Executive, 2000; Scottish Executive, 2001), these being written instructions to support the administration of medicines without direct medical assessment and prescription. These PGDs are, however, only appropriate for the administration of named medicines in a defined clinical situation when the care is consistent (NMC, 2002b).

In the UK, the prescription, supply and administration of medicines are legislated by the Medicines Act 1968, any breaches of which are liable to criminal prosecution. The legality of group protocols in line with the Medicines Act was questioned, with the result that the whole subject and process were reviewed by a DoH working party chaired by Dr June Crown (DoH, 1999a). Sections 55 (1) (b) and 58 (2) (b) of the Act require that medicines be supplied or administered on the directions of a doctor, but it was discovered that some of the protocols developed were in breach of this Act. One of the objectives of the review committee was to produce criteria, to be incorporated into group protocols, that would satisfy legal requirements. The review team definition of a group protocol is:

a specific written instruction for the supply or administration of named medicines in an identified clinical situation. It is drawn up locally by doctors, pharmacists and other appropriate professionals, and approved by the employer, advised by the relevant professional advisory committees. It applies to groups of patients or other service users who may not be individually identified before presentation for treatment.

The supply and administration of medicines under PGD protocol arrangements will be for limited aspects of care as most medicines will be provided on an individually assessed basis. New drugs under intensive monitoring are not appropriate for administration under such arrangements, nor are Schedule 4 and 5 drugs, unlicensed medications and those used in clinical trials or beyond the boundaries of their licence.

Controlled drugs cannot be administered under a PGD protocol arrangement; this includes all substances classed as Schedule 4 or 5. It is acknowledged that this restriction will prevent some aspects of advanced nursing, for example pain control and sedation practice, developing appropriately, so the Royal College of Nursing has opened discussions with the Medicines Control Agency and the Home Office in an effort to include some Schedule 4 and 5 drugs in PGD protocols in the future.

A group protocol should clearly state the clinical area and patient condition for which it is intended. The clinical criteria for patient eligibility should be included, as should criteria for the exclusion of patients from treatment under the protocol and the action to be taken in such circumstances. Staff identified to administer medicines under these arrangements should be qualified health professionals, registered with a recognized regulatory body. They should have received appropriate education and training relevant to the medications identified in the protocol. Arrangements for continued education should be stipulated in the document.

The names of medicines to be supplied and administered under the protocol, including their doses, should be listed. If a range of doses is required, the criteria for determining the dose should be available, and if more than one dose is required, the frequency of administration should be confirmed. The method or route of administration should also be identified. Arrangements for referral to a doctor should be stated, as should instructions for managing adverse events.

It is the employer's responsibility to approve the protocol to the extent that the staff identified to supply and administer medications under the PGD arrangements are indemnified. The staff involved should be provided with written evidence that they are entitled to practise under the direction of the specified PGD arrangements. Practitioners will probably be covered for indemnity under the insurance scheme of their own professional organization; this is certainly the case for Royal College of Nursing members. Practitioners who are members of other organizations should seek advice before working under group protocol arrangements. Changes to the Medicines Act as a result of the Crown review (DoH, 1999a) support the practice of incorporating properly thought out policies into practice to meet patients' needs effectively.

Risk management

Risk management initiatives have aimed to reduce the number of negligence claims within the NHS and precautions to reduce exposure to risks should be exercised at all times. Accidents and untoward treatments do, however, occur, although if all due care has been taken, nurses are unlikely to have fault found against them. Indeed, there may be particular circumstances in which exposure to risk is justified (McHale et al., 1998). If a decision were made that the benefit of having a procedure outweighed the risks, the main issue, should a claim for damages be made, would focus around the assessment and judgement of the practitioner, considering the probability of risk versus benefit. In this instance, the importance of effective documentation would clearly play a major role in determining whether the assessment was accurate and justified. Practitioners would be well advised to ensure that the assessment is documented prior to administering sedation. Also included should be information on the type and dosage of medication to be given and any accompanying care, for example supplemental oxygen or monitoring requirements. If the dosage of medication differs from that considered in the original assessment, the rationale for the alteration should be appropriately documented. This sounds time-consuming but it does allow professional judgement to be analysed and justified in the event of a complication, an adverse reaction or even a complaint.

Sedation should be administered only if appropriately trained personnel are available to provide assistance throughout the procedure, these staff being capable of monitoring the patient and initiating emergency action if required (AOMRC, 2001). Clinical risk can be minimized if one member of the care team has a defined responsibility for record-keeping and patient observation throughout the procedure (AOMRC, 2001). Despite these safety measures, an emergency may occur at any time, so it is essential that every member of the team is trained in resuscitation techniques. Life-saving equipment should be readily available and regularly checked and maintained where conscious sedation is being administered.

Clinical algorithms, guidelines and protocols

Clinical guidelines and protocols should support the clinician in decision-making. Usually based on evidence from clinical studies or expert opinion working parties, care pathways, algorithms and protocols should ensure that practice is safe and effective. However, just because a guideline exists, a court will not necessarily accept it: it must be found to be reasonable. A responsible body of opinion must recognize the algorithm guideline as advocating proper and acceptable practice.

Clinical protocols should be based on evidence of good practice and preferably supported by guidelines produced by expert professional working groups. For example, a protocol written for administration of sedation agents by a nurse in the endoscopy department should consider and support the recommendations of the British Society of Gastroenterology (1991) and the Academy of Medical Royal Colleges (2001) as minimum standards. Protocols should be dated when written and a date for review agreed. Protocols may be withdrawn if circumstances change, for example if there is an alteration in the skill mix of the nursing staff to support the advanced practitioner. Guidelines and professional judgement should be used together, always utilizing a reflective approach to evaluate practice.

Standards for record-keeping

The principles and guidelines for the recording of patient information by nurses are clearly identified by the NMC (2002c). The extent of records maintained for patients receiving sedation will vary depending on the nature and duration of the procedure. In an attempt to document objectively a description of patients' intraoperative state, scales for the assessment of intravenous conscious sedation have been developed (see Chapter 6). A tool such as that developed by Clark (1994) may require some modification if it is to be used outside the USA, but it is specific to endoscopy and does provide some useful guidelines for standards of documentation in relation to conscious sedation.

Whether or not a sedation scale is utilized, the patient's tolerance of any procedure should be recorded. Documentation should also include the patient's vital signs, the level of consciousness and all medication administered (Kidwell, 1991). In addition, any unusual events or complications and their subsequent management should be evaluated.

Advice and information

Prior to any procedure, it is useful for the patient to be prepared in advance, both from a practical point of view and to allay anxiety. Fear of the unknown can cause the patient to resist complying with unpleasant procedures, and knowing what to expect can also ensure that post-procedural care arrangements are organized.

Written information about the procedure should be given to the patient in advance so that it can be considered and any necessary arrangements made for after the procedure. Post-procedural advice should be given both verbally before the patient leaves the department and in written form, remembering to be sensitive to language and literacy variations. Instructions should include guidance on when normal activities can be resumed and what to do in the event of a complication (Fleischer, 1989).

Informed consent

When patients are offered treatments or investigative procedures, they should be given the opportunity to discuss them in a manner that provides both an understanding of the rationale for the plan of care and a simple explanation of what to expect. People have a moral and ethical right to be aware of any procedures they are to undergo and the risks to which they might be exposed (DoH, 2001); these are basic principles of informed consent. Unfortunately, these are sometimes, for many reasons, misapplied in the healthcare environment, resulting in confusion and unnecessary anxiety for patients and their families.

Although there is a legal requirement to disclose information to patients on their state of health and the risks and benefits of treatment, there will be occasions on which a decision is made to withhold information from the patient (*Sidaway* v. *Board of Governors of Bethlem Royal Hospital* 1985). This is known as 'therapeutic privilege' and is used when it is thought that a patient is unable to cope with the full details of his or her diagnosis and prognosis. The NMC supports this principle, advocating that when patients are unable or refuse to receive information about their condition, the practitioner should respect their wishes at all times, aiming to be sensitive to the needs of the individual (NMC, 2002a).

The consent forms that patients are asked to sign prior to procedures being carried out confirm only that a signature has been requested and not necessarily that the person signing the form has understood the implications of the procedure. For healthcare practitioners to be able to relinquish liability for negligence, they must be able to prove that the patient understood what the procedure entailed. In order for consent to be legally valid, the practitioner should be able to demonstrate that consent was given freely, without coercion. If a serious medical procedure such as endoscopy is to be carried out, implied consent, such as turning up for a procedure at the allotted time or having taken the prescribed bowel preparation, is not a sufficient indication that the patient understands the procedure.

An assessment should be made of the patient's capacity to understand. Most people are capable of making decisions for themselves, but when faced with new words, informed of risks and advised that a form must be signed to indicate their agreement to proceed, patients may appear confused and require further clarification. The patient is not necessarily being difficult. Patients basically need simple explanations about forthcoming procedures, what to expect and how they should prepare. It will usually be the person scheduled to carry out the procedure who will obtain the consent (NMC, 2002a). The doctor is often the one who discusses the implications of future care management plans with the patient and obtains consent for any procedures, but it is left to the nurse to provide clarification and reassurance for the patient. This is acceptable and good practice as, in times of stress and diminished cognitive function, explanations may need to be reinforced. It does not necessarily indicate that earlier discussions have not in fact taken place but is merely a mechanism to give added emphasis to explanations and understanding.

If there are reservations about a person's mental ability to understand, he or she may be assessed as mentally incompetent to give consent. English law allows such patients to be given those treatments which professionals treating the patient believe to be in his or her best interest. As far as possible, however, care strategies should be discussed with all patients, and they should be involved in the decision-making relating to their future options and investigations. When decision-making capability is a problem, guidelines from the Law Commission (1995) recommend as much patient participation as possible, ascertaining the past and present desires or preferences of the person concerned, the views of others able to act in the patient's best interests and a consideration of less invasive actions. It may also be helpful to refer the case for a second opinion.

Failure to obtain consent may lead to the patient suing for damages in the civil courts. Here, the patient will need to prove that the practitioner had a duty of care, that the duty was broken and that damage occurred as a result of the breach. With regard to consent, the two crimes seen most often in the law courts are battery, for unlawful touching, and negligence, for failing to provide sufficient information. There is currently much debate over how much information to give to patients, particularly on the extent to which procedural risks should be highlighted. The law requires patients to be informed of the nature of the procedure (*Chatterton* v. *Gerson* 1981).

It is legally acceptable to give treatment without consent in an emergency situation: the court would uphold this decision providing it could be proved that the procedure was necessary. If there is any doubt that a procedure would be against the patient's wishes, and providing there is sufficient time, advice may be sought from the court.

During the assessment and consent period, the patient should be offered an explanation of the sedation techniques available and the procedure to be carried out. Before arriving for the procedure, written instructions on the procedure and on methods of pain and anxiety control should have been given or sent (SAAD, 2000; DoH, 2001). Endoscopy departments increasingly post the patient information that includes informed consent details and discharge advice, allowing these to be considered in advance. This arrangement should always include department or named staff contact details in case further clarification is required. This facility may, however, prove to be a drain on resources as the appropriate personnel may not always be available to deal with telephone queries involving such matters as sedation techniques or risk ratios associated with the procedure.

A working party from the BSG has produced extensive guidelines for informed consent for endoscopic procedures (BSG, 1999). These include a comprehensive section advising on information that patients want or ought to know before deciding whether to consent to an investigation or treatment.

Higher-level practitioner

The *Scope of Professional Practice* (UKCC, 1992) supports the extension and expansion of role of the nurse in order more adequately and appropriately to meet patient requirements. The emergence of advanced practitioner and senior clinical nursing roles with an emphasis on responding to patients' needs has subsequently resulted in the recognition that some nurses are in a position of a higher level of practice.

The NMC does not currently define specific standards or training requirements for clinical nurse specialist and advanced practitioner roles. Employers and employees are producing a variety of job descriptions with their own emphasis and interpretation of responsibilities and educational requirements, with the result of that there is no minimum educational requirement in this area. Existing arrangements for the regulation of postregistration qualifications lack transparency and consistency. Responsibilities differ vastly from one local hospital to another, job titles being varied and misleading. This not only prevents the public making judgements about the nurse, but is also very confusing to other healthcare professionals.

The NMC now intends to clarify and update the current postregistration framework for nurses and formally to recognize nurses working at a higher level of practice. Discussions related to recording specialist practitioner qualifications on the nurses' professional register are ongoing, and the results of this debate should allow a recognition of attainment at a higher level. It is anticipated that this initiative will enable an improvement in and evaluation of standards, in addition to supporting the principle of lifelong learning, linking regulation requirements and practice developments to continuing professional education (DoH, 1999b).

The core principles of this development, as agreed by the UKCC and to be considered further by the NMC, are as follows:

1. A higher level of practice will be based on clinical competence.
2. The recognition of those working at a higher level of practice will be based on a demonstration that clinical competence has been attained, this being supported by appropriate postregistration education.
3. There will be a UK-wide standard of practice, generic to all healthcare settings.
4. The threshold for the standard will incorporate assessing, planning, implementing and reviewing practice at a higher level.
5. The focus will be competency in practice achieved through an identification of outcomes defined by the specification of clear criteria.

The NMC will in future require notification from nurses of their intention to practise at a higher level and of their wish to continue to practise at that level. It is expected that these advanced practitioners will be subjected to rigorous periodic assessment, by a specialist panel of experts, in an effort to maintain standards.

Evidence-based care

Changing the way in which care is given to ensure an incorporation of relevant scientific evidence is commonly referred to as evidence-based practice. It is a requirement of every nurse as identified by the NMC to keep up to date with developments, knowledge and competence in practice (2002a); therefore every nurse should be comfortable and familiar with approaches to analysis of evidence.

Broadly speaking, there are three categories of evidence available:

1. systematic reviews of published research;
2. individual research;
3. expert opinion or working party guidelines.

To the novice appraiser of research, it is more reliable and certainly simpler to evaluate systematic reviews and expert opinion guidelines, always remembering of course that evidence must be appraised in relation to one's own environment. Consideration should be given to how clearly the results indicate that the practice is successful, taking into account an analysis of costs and benefits.

Clinical effectiveness is about measuring the extent to which clinical actions do what they are meant to do. When determining clinical effectiveness, the first step is to find information on effective practice. Then, having found information you are comfortable with and confident of, action can be taken to incorporate this new or modified method of practice into your clinical environment. All change should of course be monitored, and, following a suitable trial period with perhaps a degree of modification along the way, the intervention should be evaluated.

Conclusion and recommendations

The legal rather than the ethical standpoint has been identified in this chapter, but the nurse should be reminded that the law is complex and at times uncertain. In clinical practice, it is important to be able to justify one's actions; accountability is about doing something because it is right, hopefully within the relevant legal system but certainly from an ethical and moral principle.

This chapter has considered some of the professional and legal aspects pertinent to the clinical practice of conscious sedation; it has never been the intention of the author to replicate all of the relevant cases in relation to healthcare law but merely to highlight some important issues. Practitioners do, however, need to be confident that they are, in their practice, maintaining as a minimum the standard identified by their professional body and they must also ensure that they practise within the legal framework. To enable professional judgement and skill to be incorporated into an environment in which uncertainty may inhibit the adherence of practice to protocols and guidelines, practitioners should be confident of their legal duties and responsibilities. The author therefore recommends this chapter as an introduction to the subject and advises readers to investigate the subject further, using books, articles and conferences identified specifically for the purpose.

Table of cases

Bolam *v*. Friern Hospital Management Committee [1957] 1 WLR 582.
Chatterton *v*. Gerson [1981] 1 All ER 574.
Sidaway *v*. Board of Governors of Bethlem Royal Hospital [1985] 1 AC 871.

References

Academy of Medical Royal Colleges (2001). Implementing and Ensuring Safe Sedation Practice for Healthcare Procedures in Adults. www.aomrc.org.uk/RCA.
British Society of Gastroenterology (1991) Recommendations for standards of sedation and patient monitoring during gastrointestinal endoscopy. Gut 32: 823–7.
British Society of Gastroenterology (1999) Guidelines for Informed Consent for Endoscopic Procedures. www.bsg.org.uk
Clark BA (1994) A new approach to assessment and documentation of conscious sedation during endoscopic examinations. Gastroenterology Nursing 16(5): 199–203.
Department of Health (1999a) Review of Prescribing, Supply and Administration of Medicines. Final Report (Crown Report). London: DoH.
Department of Health (1999b) Making a Difference: Strengthening the Nursing, Midwifery and Health Visiting Contribution to Health and Healthcare. London: DoH.
Department of Health (2001) Good Practice in Consent Implementation Guide: Consent to Examination or Treatment. London: DoH.
Fleischer D (1989) Monitoring the patient receiving conscious sedation for gastrointestinal endoscopy. Gastrointestinal Endoscopy 35: 265–7.
General Medical Council (1995) Duties of a Doctor: Guidelines from the General Medical Council. Good Medical Practice. London: GMC.
Kidwell J (1991) Nursing care of the patient receiving conscious sedation during gastrointestinal procedures. Gastroenterology Nursing 13(3): 134–9.
Law Commission (1995) Mental Incapacity. Law Commission Report No. 231. London: HMSO.
McHale J, Tingle J, Pey
sner J (1998) Law and Nursing. Oxford: Butterworth-Heinemann.
Montgomery J (1992) Doctors' handmaidens: the legal contribution. In: McVeigh S, Whelar S (eds) Law, Health and Medical Regulation. Aldershot: Dartmouth.

National Assembly for Wales (2000) Review of Prescribing, Supply and Administration of Medicines by Health Professionals under Patient Group Directions. Cardiff: NAW.

National Health Service Executive (2000) Patient Group Directions (England Only). Leeds: NHSE.

Nursing and Midwifery Council (2002a) Code of Professional Conduct. London: NMC.

Nursing and Midwifery Council (2002b) Guidelines for the Administration of Medicines. London: NMC.

Nursing and Midwifery Council (2002c) Guidelines for Records and Record-keeping. London: NMC.

Scottish Executive (Health Department) (2001) Patient Group Directions. Edinburgh: SE.

Society for the Advancement of Anaesthesia in Dentistry (2000). Standards in Conscious Sedation in Dentistry: The Report of an Independent Working Group Produced by the Society for the Advancement of Anaesthesia in Dentistry. www.saaduk/org/sedbooklet.

United Kingdom Central Council for Nursing, Midwifery and Health Visiting (1992) Scope of Professional Practice. London: UKCC.

United Kingdom Central Council for Nursing, Midwifery and Health Visiting (1998) Higher Level Practice (Specialist Practice Project-Phase 11) cc/98/19. London: UKCC.

Index

149